NUTRITION AND THE EYES

HOW TO KEEP YOUR EYES HEALTHY NATURALLY

VOLUME II

By
Bill Sardi

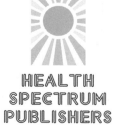

HEALTH
SPECTRUM
PUBLISHERS

Sardi, Bill
    Nutrition and The Eyes

Includes index
1. Nutrition and human vision. 2. Nutrition— therapeutic use.

ISBN 1-885919-47-6

This book has been typeset to aid the visually impaired.

Health Spectrum Publishers
8851 Central Avenue, G-620
Montclair, CA. 91763

NUTRITION AND THE EYES
TABLE OF CONTENTS
VOLUME II

THE HUMAN EYE

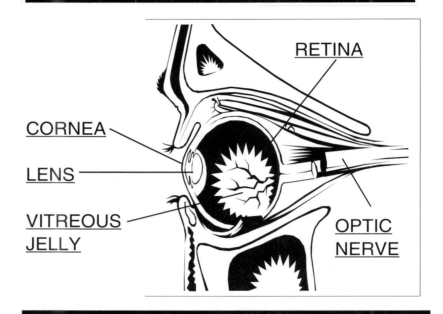

RETINA

CORNEA

LENS

VITREOUS JELLY

OPTIC NERVE

WHERE EYE DISEASE OCCURS

LOCATION	KEY EYE DISORDERS
CORNEA	DRY EYE HERPES EYE INFECTIONS KERATOCONUS PTERYGIUM
LENS	PRESBYOPIA CATARACTS
VITREOUS	FLOATERS VITREOUS DETACHMENT
RETINA	MACULAR DEGENERATION RETINITIS PIGMENTOSA DIABETIC RETINOPATHY
OPTIC NERVE	GLAUCOMA

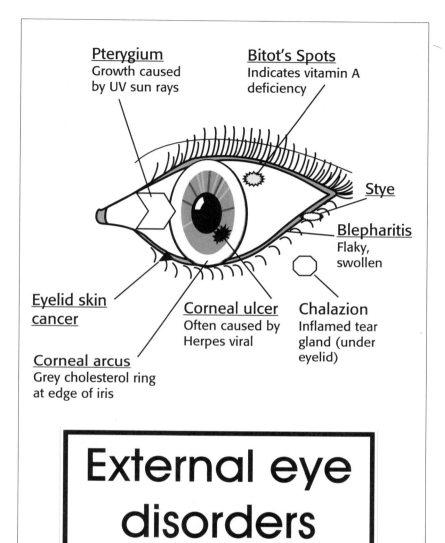

Pterygium
Growth caused
by UV sun rays

Bitot's Spots
Indicates vitamin A
deficiency

Stye

Blepharitis
Flaky,
swollen

Eyelid skin cancer

Corneal ulcer
Often caused by
Herpes viral

Chalazion
Inflamed tear
gland (under
eyelid)

Corneal arcus
Grey cholesterol ring
at edge of iris

External eye disorders

GENERAL DISCLAIMER
Please Read

The information in this book cannot substitute for periodic eye examinations. While self-care and prevention should be encouraged, most eye disorders cannot be self-detected in their early stages when treatment or preventive measures work best to preserve sight. The information in this book is taken from the medical literature. Readers are encouraged to share this information with their own eye physician and to seek other sources of information concerning eye problems. Readers are also encouraged to tell their eye physician that they believe in preventive medicine and that they wish to practice some of the measures in this book under the physician's supervision.

The nutritional recommendations in this text are general in nature and not intended for every patient since the particular medical history, allergies and current prescription drug use are unknown to the author. Do not stop taking any vitamin or medication your doctor has prescribed without consultation. The author is not a physician. The reader should not consider the educational information in this text as the practice of medicine.

The author has attempted to provide the latest medical data available. However, there may be errors of omission or typesetting. Therefore the reader is encouraged to seek other sources of information and the wise counsel of their physician before embarking upon changes in lifestyle or nutrition.

The author and publisher shall bear neither liability nor responsibility to any person or entity with respect to any loss or damage caused, or alleged to be caused, directly or indirectly by the information contained in this book.

If you do not wish to be bound by the above, you may return this book to the publisher for a full refund.

CROSS REFERENCE DIRECTORY OF EYE TOPICS		
If you have....	**Also read .....**	**Located in .....**
Eye allergy	Dry eye Digestive problems	Volume I Volume II
Blepharitis	Eye allergy	Volume I
Blepharospasm	Dry eye	Volume I
Cataracts	Sunglasses Uveitis Side effects of drugs Sugar cataracts Smoking and the eyes	Volume II Volume III Volume II Volume III Volume II
Computer eyestrain	Dry eye Eye allergy	Volume I Volume I
Corneal transplant	Herpes eye infections	Volume III
Diabetes	Cataracts Circulatory disorders	Volume I Volume II
Driver vision	Cataracts Night vision	Volume I Volume III
Droopy eyelids	Smoking & the eyes	Volume II
Eyelid skin cancer	Sunglasses	Volume II
Flashes and floaters	Retinal detachment	Volume II
Glaucoma	Circulatory disorders	Volume II
Keratoconus	Eye allergy	Volume I
Macular degeneration	Circulatory disorders	Volume II
Migraine	Circulatory disorders Eye Allergy Artificial sweeteners Digestion	Volume II Volume I Volume II Volume II

CROSS REFERENCE DIRECTORY		
Myopia	**Retinal detachment**	**Volume II**
Night vision	Retinitis pigmentosa	Volume II
Pterygium	Sunlight & sunglasses	Volume II
Retinal detachment	Myopia	Volume I
Retinitis pigmentosa	Night vision Drug side effects	Volume II Volume II
Ocular rosacea	Digestion & the eyes	Volume II
Sjogrens' syndrome	Dry eyes Digestion & the eyes	Volume I Volume II
Trichaisis	Blepharitis	Volume I

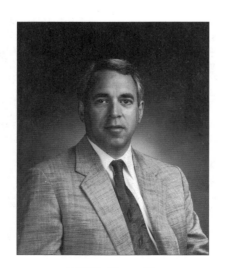

Bill Sardi

About The Author

Bill Sardi has spent the past 15 years in the eye care field and has visited over 2000 ophthalmologist's offices. He has served as consultant to companies in the eye care field, has conducted numerous surveys of physicians and patients, authored two books, lectured at various professional meetings, and wrote a documentary report on cataract care for the Society of Geriatric Ophthalmology. An advocate for patients, Bill's collection of over 3000 scientific reports has culminated in NUTRITION AND THE EYES, the most authoritative text of its kind. This book opens a whole new era of preventive eye care.

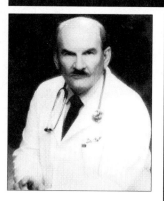

Donald J. Carrow M.D.
Talk Radio's Medical Maverick

Foreward

Answering questions about health and nutrition, as I do weekly on a nationwide radio talk show, I know the most frequently asked questions concern the eyes. When I hear people's voices on the telephone who have eye problems I can hear the desperation and fear in their voices. If there is a subgroup of people who are the most willing to give nutrition a try it is adults who have been told their eye condition is hopeless.

I can say that nutritional medicine gives people more than just hope. It also provides a way of getting at eye diseases (in fact all diseases) at the molecular level where they begin. The feared enemy of the cells in the body is oxidation. This is a normal process that gets the upper hand when disease occurs. It can be countered with an array of antioxidants — such as vitamin E, vitamin C, carotenes, coenzyme Q10, selenium and the family of bioflavonoids (quercetin, ginkgo biloba, bilberry and others.) Each of the 33 eye disorders in this book includes nutritional recommendations centered around antioxidants.

Are there safe and effective nutritional "cures" for many common eye disorders? Not only does this book document that fact but numerous times I have observed cloudy cataracts that have cleared, cases of macular degeneration that have improved, and cases of glaucoma that have been controlled following a nutritional regimen. It is sad that more physicians are not familiar with these approaches to ocular disorders.

You will likely read the sections of this book that pertain to your eye problems. Don't overlook many other sections. Use the handy cross-reference guide to other related conditions. For example, if you have glaucoma you must read the chapter on circulatory problems. If you have ocular rosacea, Sjogrens' syndrome, or any optic nerve problem you need to read the chapter on digestive disorders.

If you are like most people you don't really want to know as much about what causes your particular eye problem as you do about how to fix it. You will probably flip to the back pages of the chapter that covers your eye problem and read which nutrients you need to take. After you have learned which nutrients may be helpful for your condition read the handy guide to vitamins and nutritional products in the accompanying supplement. This will give you a better idea of which brands of nutritional supplements may be helpful for your condition.

Keep in mind, this book doesn't promise anyone instant cures nor that they will get their sight back. But, again, there is good reason to follow the nutritional regimens outlined herein.

For skeptical health professionals who read this book, I suggest looking up at least some of the 700+ references listed to gain a personal understanding of the benefits of nutritional medicine.

When you finish reading the section of this book that pertains to your eye problem I would encourage you to share this book with others.

This book is part of a revolution taking place in medicine today. Patients are demanding more preventive and nutritional approaches to health problems. The popularity of our radio talk show proves that people prefer health care over disease care.

While you are encouraged to ask your physician about the nutritional regimens in this book, your eye doctor will most likely be unfamiliar with this information. Just remember, every time you ask doctors about nutritional approaches to health problems you let them know that the public is seeking this brand of medicine. It won't take long for doctors to realize, if they want to keep their patients, that they will need to improve their knowledge about nutrition.

Donald Carrow M.D.
"Here's To Your Health" radio show
Tampa, Florida

1

Introduction

This book provides information to help you:

Prevent eye disorders before they begin.

Delay the progress or even reverse the course of an eye disorder once it has been detected.

Preserve your remaining vision if some sight has already been lost.

Many people avoid eye doctors because "no news is good news." Nobody wants to be told they are going blind. Blindness is the most feared of handicaps.[1] Fear breeds on a lack of information. The good news contained within the pages of this book is that chronic eye problems can be overcome by practicing preventive medicine at home.

The fearful are more likely to turn to alternative medical treatments to cure their ailments. In 1990 American adults spent over $10 billion out of their own pocket for alternative medical treatments ranging from vitamin therapy, acupuncture, iridology, eye exercises, etc. Fear can also leave patients open to the suggestion of any "cure" to keep from losing sight. This book should help clear up many myths about the eyes.

The limits of medical research

Recognize that medical reports are derived from groups of people. This means, if you practice preventive measures, you will significantly reduce the odds that you will develop eye problems. Medical reports don't necessarily apply to your particular eye problem.

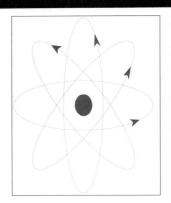

An unpaired electron whirling around a molecule is known as a free radical. Free radicals oxidize or destroy cells within the body. Antioxidants counter the free radicals and thus help to preserve health.

Because of the many breakthroughs in treating cataracts with lens implants and the use of lasers to treat retinal conditions and glaucoma, physicians have been distracted from the many advancements occurring in nutritional medicine. Patients frequently bring news clippings about nutritional cures for eye disorders to their eye doctor. Physicians don't have the time to investigate each of these reports so they are usually dismissed. Medical schools do not provide physicians with sufficient training about nutrition.

Nutrition: How it works

The food chain has changed dramatically since the 1930's. America eats more processed foods now. The cooking and canning of foods destroys valuable nutrients. The entire nutrient load of a 2500 calorie meal amounts to only a few small granules.

Eating a well balanced diet that contains all of the food groups (meat, dairy, grains and vegetables) still does not provide optimal levels of nutrients required to prevent disease.

Older Americans have 10 times more eye problems than younger aged adults. Nutritional requirements for older adults are greater than for those of younger age.

America is becoming enlightened about the role of nutrition in preventing disease. Time Magazine made vitamins a front page story in a recent issue.

Many health problems have been eliminated by nutrition.

⇒ Rickets has vanished with inclusion of vitamin D in milk.

⇒ Beri beri has been eradicated with thiamine (vitamin B1).

⇒ Scurvy has been erased with vitamin C.

⇒ Many doctors now recommend folic acid to prevent birth abnormalities among pregnant women.

⇒ Niacin is used to flush out cholesterol.

⇒ Vitamin E is recommended to reduce the risk of heart attack.

⇒ Vitamin B6 reduces the symptoms of carpal tunnel syndrome.

⇒ Vitamin B12 reduces fatigue among geriatric patients.

⇒ Magnesium overcomes heart spasm.

⇒ Calcium reverses osteoporosis.

⇒ Fiber helps to control blood sugar and improve digestion.

⇒ Multiple antioxidant nutrients are prescribed to aid in healing burns or to prevent debilitation from AIDS.

⇒ Eye surgeons add glutathione, an antioxidant, to the fluids they use to irrigate the eyes during eye surgery.

⇒ The National Cancer Institute and the American Heart Association now recommend foods and nutrients high in beta carotene, vitamin C and vitamin E to reduce risks of heart disease and cancer.

⇒ Dermatologists use Retin-A, a derivative of vitamin A, to reverse skin aging.

It looks like vitamins are becoming very popular with doctors!

The power of antioxidants

Diseases start at the cellular level. A process called oxidation is believed to be involved in most forms of cellular destruction. Antioxidants are the antidote to oxidation. The cells of the body can be destroyed when a single unpaired electron spinning around an oxygen atom seeks to find a mate. These are known as "free radicals," atomic sized destroyers on a "kamikaze" mission.

Antioxidants work like a "pac man," counteracting the oxidation process. **The antioxidants "chew up" the free radicals.** The body makes some of its own antioxidants, such as glutathione, super oxide dismutase, catalase and coenzyme Q10. Nutrients such as selenium, riboflavin, zinc and cysteine are needed to help the body produce these antioxidant enzymes. Some antioxidants are derived from the diet, such as vitamin C, vitamin E, vitamin A, bioflavonoids, selenium, and many others.

All human disease is now believed to have some relationship with free radicals and oxidation.[2] The oxidation process has long been studied within the human eye. Researchers have demonstrated that oxidation is involved in the development of virtually all eye disorders, including cataracts, retinal disease and glaucoma.[3]

Certain structures of the body exhibit accelerated oxidation. The lungs exchange oxygen with carbon dioxide, so there is a plentiful supply of oxygen molecules for the oxidation process in the lungs. Ultraviolet sun rays promote oxidation, and the eyelids, cornea, sclera, iris, lens, vitreous and retina of the eye are exposed to daily dosages of UV rays. The cornea and lens of the eye focus or intensify UV rays on the retina.

The fluid that fills the front of the eye (called the aqueous) has one of the highest levels of vitamin C in the body. The retina at the back of the eye is supplied with antioxidant nutrients from the blood stream. When oxidation overwhelms the antioxidants, cells are destroyed.

With age the body produces fewer of its own antioxidants. Over time, the oxidation process can slowly weaken the tissues of the body and eventually affect vision.

Stare directly at the midday sun and the UV rays can burn or "oxidize" retinal cells at the back of the eyes in a few minutes, resulting in loss of central vision. Likewise, the destruction of retinal cells can occur slowly over many years, from low levels of sunlight or from a gradual reduction in the antioxidant defense system. The diminished level of antioxidants in the eyes with advancing age is believed to be the major factor in the weakening of sight in the later years.

The missing nutrient: Essential fatty acids

Every bit as important as are antioxidants to the maintenance of eye health are omega-3 fats, found in fish oil and in flax seed.

Because Americans consume 100% more saturated fats and cholesterol than Americans who lived over 100 years ago,[4] a host of new diseases have begun to plague modern man. Add to those saturated fats the new "plastic" man-made fats found in margarines, egg substitutes, and baked goods, and it's easy to see why our blood vessels are lined with cholesterol and fats that lead to cardiovascular and heart disease, as well as a host of age-related eye problems like macular degeneration, retinal vein occlusion, glaucoma, temporal arteritis, and all of the neovascular (oxygen-starved) eye disorders.

It doesn't take a rocket scientist to realize that the tiny blood vessels located in the eyes can become clogged with fats that result in eye problems before health maladies become evident elsewhere in the body.

Dr. Donald Rudin MD, in his book THE OMEGA-3 PHENOMENON (Rawson Associates, New York 1987), says omega-3 oils, found in cold-climate plants and fish, are a "nutritional missing link." These omega-3 oils are commonly found in flax seed, soy, walnuts, wheat germ, chestnuts, northern beans and fish such as cod, salmon, tuna and mackerel.

Americans are developing an aversion to fats, but there are "good" fats that promote health. The omega-3 variety of fats are unsaturated, that is, they still remain liquid at room temperature, whereas saturated fats turn hard. Omega-3 fats can be likened to nature's "anti-freeze" for humans.

These omega-3 fats help to regulate a number of functions in the body, including regulation of eye pressure, constriction of blood vessels, thinning of the blood, moistening the skin and eyes, relieving spasms (eyelids, muscles, etc.), reducing sun sensitivity, reducing cholesterol, relieving symptoms of arthritis, and boosting the immune system.

The American diet is filled with saturated oils in hamburgers, fried foods, greasy sandwiches, and with advancing age, Americans are paying for this over-consumption of saturated fats with their eyesight.

It's important to understand that these omega-3 oils, as essential as they are for health maintenance, need to be combined with the antioxidants. Oils turn rancid, a destructive process called lipid peroxidation within the body. But the antioxidants protect the oils from spoilage. Combined together, through proper diet or nutritional supplements, antioxidants and omega-3 oils can help to prolong years of health and good vision.

REFERENCES

[1] "The worst disability that could happen," National Eye Health Education Program, National Institutes of Health. undated monograph.
[2] Voelker R., "Radical approaches: is widespread testing and treatment for oxidative injuries coming soon?," Journal American Medical Association 270: 2024, November 3, 1993.
[3] Taylor A., Jacques P.F., Dorey K.C., "Oxidation and aging: Impact on vision," Submitted for publication, Tufts University USDA Human Nutrition Research Center on Aging, 1993.
[4] Erasmus U., FATS AND OILS, Alive Books, Vancouver, 1986, p. 149.

Quick facts

<u>Part of the eye affected.</u> Center of the retina (macula)

<u>Typical age of onset.</u> Past the sixth decade of life

<u>Risk factors.</u> Blue eyes, sun exposure, aging spots on the retina (drusen), high fat diet, smoking.

<u>Modern treatment.</u> Only a small number of patients can be treated with laser.

<u>Preventive measures:</u> UV-blocking sunglasses, blood thinners, anti-vasospasm agents (calcium channel blockers), very low fat and cholesterol diet, antioxidant nutritional supplements, smoking cessation, daily exercise.

<u>Questions to ask your eye doctor:</u>

Do I have aging spots (drusen) at the back of my eyes?
Can this disease be prevented?

2
MACULAR DEGENERATION
(Also called aging retinal disease)

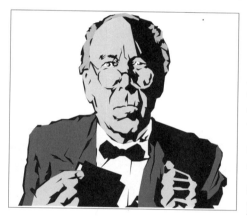

Franklin is relatively healthy for an octogenarian. He does his 50 pushups every morning and takes his vitamins with breakfast. He enjoys swimming and wants to go on living another decade or two. His greatest frustration is that he has lost some of his central vision and he can't read books anymore. He can't understand why he is so healthy but has lost some of his sight. His trusted eye physician tells him there is nothing he can do about the vision he has lost. His wife reads a newspaper clipping to him about injections of interferon that could possibly help cure his loss of sight. Franklin flies across the country to find out about the injections. He is disappointed. The injections aren't helpful for his type of retinal disease. Franklin says he would travel anyplace on earth if he could get his vision back. He eagerly awaits any scientific breakthrough.

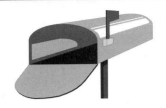

Mail bag

I was recently diagnosed with macular degeneration which was a complete surprise and unwelcome surprise to me. The ophthalmologist suggested I take vitamins. Will this be helpful?

M.M.
Redding, California

I am getting macular degeneration. I'm taking nutrients and going to a nutritional chiropractor. It seems to be helping a little. Are there any eye drops or nutrients you might suggest?

A.T.
W. Mifflin,
Pennsylvania

What is macular degeneration?

Macular degeneration, usually age-related, is defined as a progressive deterioration of the central retina called the macula.

Macular degeneration results in loss of central vision, occurring more frequently after age 65. There are several varieties of this eye disorder divided into what doctors call the "wet" and "dry" forms. The vast majority of cases are slow-progressing, while less than 10 percent are fast-progressing.

Macular degeneration involves the one millimeter area of the central retina used for reading vision; thus it robs one of central reading vision. This eye disorder is also called aging retinal disease.

What are the misconceptions about macular degeneration?

1. Despite what is said about cataracts and glaucoma robbing people of their sight, it is macular degeneration that is the fastest growing cause of legal blindness in the U.S. with over 15 million affected.[1]

2. Macular degeneration does not lead to total blindness. Side vision is unimpaired. Many older adults are fearful they will go totally blind from this eye disorder.

3. Laser treatment is only applicable to a small number of patients who have macular degeneration and does not improve nor preserve sight. While there are many new developments in the treatment of macular degeneration once sight has deteriorated none offer complete restoration of sight. Many macular disease patients eagerly hope they will regain the vision of their youth with some new-found "cure."

Laser treatment is used to arrest the advancement of the fast-progressing form of macular degeneration. Eye surgeons are having second thoughts about the benefits of laser treatment for macular degeneration (see below). Laser treatment does not improve vision. In some selected cases laser treatment may slow down the progression of this disease.

4. Confusion over the types of macular degeneration.

Many people are confused to hear there are two varieties of macular degeneration, "wet" and "dry." The less common "wet" form of the disease refers to new unwanted blood vessels that form and begin to progress towards the macula or visual center of the eye. The "wet" form progresses so fast that it can damage vision within a matter of days. The "wet" form of macular degeneration results when oxygen supply to the retina is blocked causing neovascularization (new blood vessel formation). The "dry" form of the disease refers to the common form that progresses slowly as a result of vascular (blood vessel disease), daily bombardment by solar ultraviolet rays and reduced levels of antioxidants.

How many have macular degeneration?

The typical person with aging retinal disease is over age 70, has blue eyes, has a family history of the disease, and may have a history of tobacco use. This person has likely spent a lot of time in the sun during his/her lifetime, and has some aging changes in the skin caused by sunlight, and has aging spots at the back of their eyes.

It is estimated that macular degeneration only accounts for 116,000 cases of legal blindness in the U.S. and 16,000 new cases are reported each year.[2] The actual number of cases is likely much larger because most cases go unreported.

The odds that one will develop macular degeneration increase with age, especially after age 65. Only 1.6 percent of adults age 52-64 have macular degeneration, but between age 65-74 this increases to 11 percent. Between age 75-85, nearly 28 percent have problems with their central vision from this disease.[3]

Macular degeneration usually begins in one eye. Four years after this eye disorder has been detected in the first eye, 23 percent of patients will develop a weak retina in their second eye.[4]

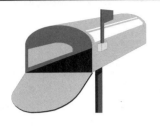

Mail Bag

The doctor calls it macular degeneration. He gave me a sample bottle of vitamins and told me I would have to live the rest of my life with poor vision. What do I do now?

B.B.
Frankfort, Indiana

What is it like to have macular degeneration?

A medical doctor writes of his personal experience with macular degeneration:

"If people could be aware of what types of images they would see when they have macular degeneration, it might help them understand and find out sooner about the problem. I had no idea of what sorts of images I was going to see or why straight lines were crooked; now I know. Outlines become wavy. There are no longer hard edges to things but a blending of the object into surrounding space. Parts of the telephone and electric lines appear fuzzy, foggy, or crooked. If I look straight ahead at a landscape, shapes are distorted at the periphery and in the center it's foggy. When I look at a person's face I can see an indistinct, steamy shape. Underneath the face is a white shirt, and on top of it is a hat. I can't recognize anyone.
  --- Comments by Terrence C. Billings, M.D., at age 72.[5]

People with aging retinal disease wish there was something more that could be done for their vision and continually ask if there is any hope they will get their central vision back. With macular degeneration one can't see a computer screen easily, read a book, watch TV, recognize faces, drive an automobile, or enjoy most hobbies. It is a frustrating visual disorder.

Most people hear of breakthroughs in the treatment of macular disease and eagerly try them for awhile, then months later give up hope that these measures will ever help their sight. Interferon injections, zinc supplements, magnifying goggles, and retinal transplants are among the "cures" that people read about in the newspapers. This book should help you understand if their is any validity to the claims that these treatments work.

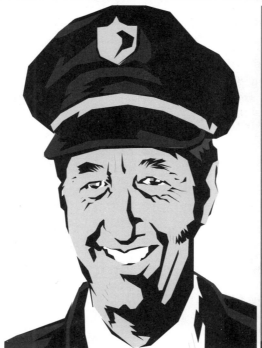 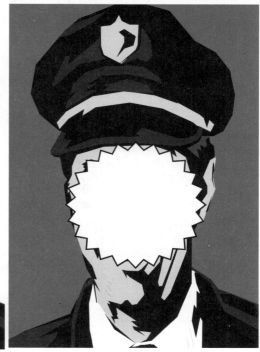

NORMAL VISION: The entire scene is visible .

MACULAR DEGENERATION: Central vision is obscured. There is difficulty reading and recognizing faces.

How well can a person see with macular degeneration?

In a study of macular disease patients:[6]

Only 29 percent could read Reader's Digest titles.

48 percent could read a clock from 6 feet.

30 percent could not correctly identify colors, especially grey and tan.

32 percent could not identify common household products, such labels on cereal boxes and catsup bottles.

74 percent could not properly visualize the facial expression on photos.

When the two types of macular degeneration are compared, 84 percent of patients with the fast progressing "wet" form are legally blind while only 12 percent of patients with the common "dry" form are legally blind.[7]

Note: if vision is 20/200 or worse in the best eye, this is classified as being legal blindness. Apply for an identification card from the American Foundation for the Blind. This card identifies partially sighted persons and qualifies them for various benefits, tax deductions, and other privileges. See the back of this book for information.

Quick home eye test for macular degeneration

While not a foolproof test, this is how the eyes can be tested for early stages of macular degeneration. If over age 65, this test is important to take daily.

Look at something that is straight, like a telephone pole, edge of a doorway or reading material, and with glasses on, close or cover one eye. Test the other eye in a similar manner. If the straight lines look wavy, crooked or different you may have a weak retina. Attempt to determine if your vision is equally bright on both sides. If it isn't, it's time to call an eye doctor for an appointment.

Slower reading speed after age 65 is another tell-tale sign of early macular degeneration.[8] If it takes your eyes a prolonged period of time to adapt after entering a room from the bright outdoors, this may be another sign of macular degeneration.[9]

What is the modern treatment for macular degeneration?

Macular degeneration patients are discouraged when they hear that there is no effective treatment for this disease.

Widely reported claims that Interferon injections may help this condition have led to a very expensive experiment for many patients, all for naught. The Interferon injections have only been

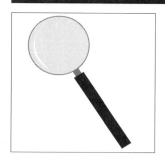

Magnifiers can be helpful for reading

reported to help patients with the less common "wet" form of the disease[10] and recent reports question the effectiveness of this treatment altogether.[11,12]

There is __no__ surgical or laser treatment for the common type of retinal disease.

A National Eye Institute report indicates laser treatment initially worsens vision among patients who have the "wet" form of macular degeneration and that the benefits of laser treatment only become apparent after a year or more when compared to patients who did not undergo treatment.[13] A recent report stated that *"overly optimistic laser treatment prophecies of the last two decades have, in reality, not been fulfilled for exudative ("wet") age-related macular disease. Despite promising expectations, it is now increasingly evident that laser treatment will not significantly reduce the severe visual loss experienced by most patients with this macular disease.... Preventive measures, such as nutritional supplements and light filtration, should also be investigated in the hope of decelerating progressive, atrophic degeneration and perhaps of reducing the conversion rate from nonexudative ("dry") to exudative ("wet") disease."*[14]

Can magnifiers help improve sight?

Macular degeneration patients need light for reading to be twice as bright as that found in the average home or office.[15] High wattage incandescent lamps in the home are recommended.

Yellow, orange and brown sunglasses, preferably of the wrap-around type, have been shown to improve vision outdoors for macular disease patients. Indoors, some patients find yellow lenses may be of help.[16]

For reading, in one study only 14 percent of macular degeneration patients could read newsprint under proper lighting conditions. When magnifiers were properly used, 92 percent of the patients were able to read the newspaper. Magnifiers of 5X power or less were most preferred, with 6X-9X power also helpful.[17] By doubling the wattage of light bulbs, better illumination can improve the reading speed of macular degeneration patients.[18]

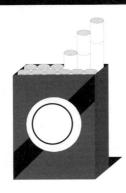

Smoking increases the risk of developing macular degeneration by 2.5 times. Smokers develop macular degeneration seven years sooner than non-smokers.

Researchers at the Johns Hopkins Wilmer Eye Institute in Baltimore, Maryland, in conjunction with the National Aeronautics and Space Administration, are developing special "wrap around" electronic vision enhancers for macular disease patients. Two miniature TV screens are built into the goggles and will help macular disease patients visualize objects while they move about.[19]

When does macular degeneration begin?

Long before one becomes aware of the disease the macula of the eye begins to deteriorate. In normal individuals the macula begins to deteriorate from youth through the age of 30 years; it appears to accelerate again after age 50. Aging spots gradually appear on the retina from age 30 to 60 and more rapidly thereafter.[20] Prevention should begin early in life to delay or avoid this common eye disorder.

Does smoking cause macular degeneration?

Compared to non-smokers, smokers who inhale have been found to have a 2.5 times increased risk of developing macular degeneration during their lifetime.[21] Smokers have been shown to develop macular degeneration in one eye at an average age of 64, non-smokers by at age 71.[22] You can buy yourself seven more years of good sight by avoiding tobacco.

It should be noted that every cigarette smoked robs the body of 25 milligrams of vitamin C. Normally the body has a pool of vitamin C equal to 2-3 grams (2,000-3,000 milligrams) which can be maintained by daily intake of at least 100 milligrams in a supplement or by diet. Decreased amounts of vitamin C may make the retina of the human eye prone to damage by sunlight.[23,24]

Smokers also have increased lipid (fats and cholesterol) levels which can block the blood vessels that carry nutrients to the retina.

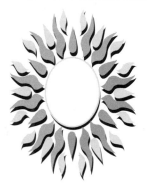

Does sunlight cause macular degeneration?

The evidence that sunlight, particularly ultraviolet and blue-violet sun rays, promotes the development of macular degeneration is overwhelming. Despite convincing evidence researchers continue to debate over which sun rays are involved with the fastest growing cause of legal blindness in the U.S.

Macular degeneration is caused by multiple factors. Sunlight is a primary or additive factor. Here is the evidence for the sunlight theory of macular degeneration.

Both the skin and the eyes are exposed to the sun. Age changes in the skin caused by sunlight are more common among people who have macular degeneration.[25]

When people develop cloudy cataracts, retinas are protected from the damaging rays of the sun. Among patients over age 60, those who develop cloudy cataracts are twice as likely NOT to develop macular degeneration as those who had no cataracts.[26] A man who lived with a traumatic cataract in one eye for 60 years developed macular degeneration in his other eye and at the age of 81 lost his sight due to hemorrhage. When eye surgeons removed the cataract in an attempt to restore sight in his eye, they observed the retina in that eye was remarkably healthy. The retina that had been shielded from sun rays by a cloudy cataract throughout the majority of this man's life showed no signs of macular degeneration.[27]

When researchers examined the eyes of fishermen, they linked their exposure to ultraviolet and blue-violet sun rays in their later years of life to the development of macular degeneration.[28]

Nearly 5000 adults age 43-84 years who lived in Beaver Dam, Wisconsin, were examined over a period from 1987 through 1990 for early signs of macular degeneration. Adults who spent more time outdoors in summer were twice as likely to develop macular disease. Those individuals who habitually wore hats and sunglasses were 40 percent less likely to develop early signs of the

What causes macular degeneration?

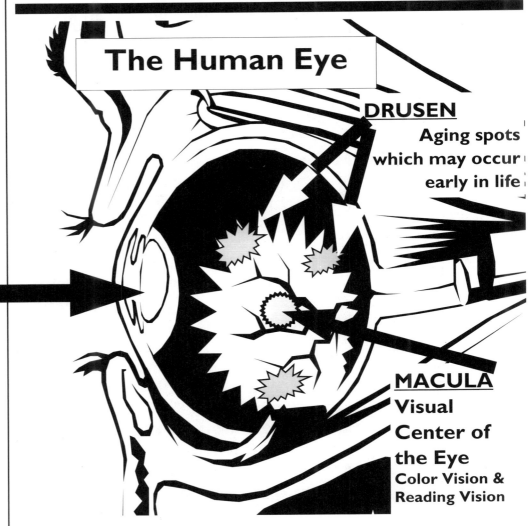

The Human Eye

DRUSEN
Aging spots which may occur early in life

MACULA
Visual Center of the Eye
Color Vision & Reading Vision

SUN LIGHT

Ultraviolet and blue-violet sun rays bombard the retina over a lifetime and accelerate aging changes in the retina.

Tiny blood vessels at the back of the eyes become progressively clogged with fats, blood clots and calcifications, starving the retina of needed oxygen and nutrition (antioxidants).

disease. Men were shown to be at an increased risk of macular degeneration. Researchers believe that women spend more time indoors and may thus have protected themselves from developing macular disease.[29]

During World War II, military personnel stationed on a tropical island and worked outdoors for four months or longer, exhibited early changes of their retinas similar to those seen in macular degeneration. These aging changes were not observed among military personnel who worked indoors.[30]

South African blacks over age 65 have more melanin pigment in their retinas which protects their eyes from sunlight damage. They have only a 1 percent incidence of macular degeneration.[31]

While the retinas of most adults over age 30 are exposed to only small amounts of UV-A and UV-B sun rays, it has been shown that a minimal amount of UV-A[32] and UV-B sun rays can damage retinal cells.

When cataracts are removed from human eyes, the amount of solar energy reaching the retina increases dramatically. It has been shown that the aging of the macula increases more rapidly following cataract surgery. In a five-year period, the retinas of patients who had cataracts removed showed accelerated aging equivalent to 30 years of normal aging.[33]

There has been some argument over which sun rays are the primary cause of macular degeneration. After age 30 or thereabouts, the natural lens of the eye discolors and blocks out nearly all UV rays from reaching the retina. However retinal light receptor cells can be damaged by blue-violet light rays.[34] This may explain why some studies have not shown a link between UV exposure and macular degeneration.[35]

The more UV and blue-violet sun rays that reach the retina of the eye, the greater the chance of developing macular degeneration. Patients with dense cataracts have only a 50 percent increased risk of developing macular disease; among those individuals who have mild cataracts, where more UV rays are permitted to reach the retina, there is an 80 percent increased risk of macular disease. **Among persons who have cataracts**

removed, the risk of macular disease increases by 200 percent. The more sun rays that reached the retina, the greater the risk of developing macular disease.[36]

Numerous experts have proposed that sunlight is a major cause of macular degeneration.[37,38] Richard W. Young, Ph.D., professor emeritus from the Jules Stein Eye Institute in Los Angeles, reveals that macular degeneration begins in the part of the retina exposed to the focused rays of the sun. He reports that blue-violet sun rays penetrate deeper into eye tissues and promote the development of garbage deposits (drusen), the hallmark sign of macular degeneration, that weaken the retina.[39] **To prevent loss of sight in the later years of life, Dr. Young advocates UV and blue-violet light protection for all persons from early youth.**

Researchers at Emory University exposed retinal photoreceptor cells in animals to 13-18 minutes of blue light rays; all of the eyes showed light damage. When blue light was filtered out only 20 percent of the eyes were burned.[40]

Despite all of the evidence presented that ultraviolet and blue-violet solar radiation promotes the development of macular degeneration, many eye doctors are confused over this issue and claim there isn't enough proof yet to link sun rays with retinal deterioration. It's up to the reader to make his or her own decision here.

There are lifetime time-windows of vulnerability in the development of macular degeneration. The retinas of the eyes are subject to continual daily bombardment of ultraviolet and blue-violet solar radiation. These can gradually bring out degenerative changes in retinal tissues, particularly after age 50 when the protective melanin pigment is slowly lost and the natural antioxidant defenses of the eyes (glutathione, super oxide dismutase, catalase) are reduced.

More UV-B and UV-A sun rays reach the retinas of youngsters because the lenses of their eyes are more transparent to harmful sun rays. Thus aging spots can be seen in the retinas of children as early as the second decade of life.[41] The fact that 97% of Americans will live into their eighth decade of life means that the lifetime exposure to unfiltered ultraviolet and blue-violet sun rays may accelerate aging of the retina and eventually affect vision.

The vulnerable time windows for solar radiation damage to the retina occur before the third decade of life, when the eye is more transparent to harmful sun rays, and after age 50 when the protective melanin and antioxidants begin to dissipate. The fact that older Americans migrate to sunny areas during their retirement years exacerbates this condition.

From youth, the habitual use of wide brimmed hats and wrap-around sun goggles is advised. The fact that it only takes one photon (one watt of light divided by one million = one photon) of UV-B sunlight to damage a retinal cell means most common sunglasses do not provide sufficient protection for the eyes. An estimated 7-40 percent of unfiltered sun rays enter the eyes while wearing conventional sunglasses.[42]

A good pair of sunglasses should block out 100 percent of the UV-A and UV-B sun rays, and filter out at least 85 percent of the blue-violet sun rays.

The fact that an estimated 40 percent of sunglasses are mislabelled on store shelves, and that the FDA is tardy in invoking and enforcing sunglass labelling laws, further frustrates the efforts to prevent macular degeneration.

While cataract lens implants do contain UV filters, eye surgeons have been mistakenly led to believe the retinas of cataract patients are completely protected from UV. Post-cataract surgery patients should wear UV-blue filtering sunglasses and take a safety dose of antioxidants every remaining day of their life.

Do antioxidants prevent macular degeneration?

Again, the evidence that antioxidants can delay or prevent the advancement of macular degeneration is overwhelming. Literally hundreds of research articles point to the fact that nutritional factors play an important role in protecting the retina.[43]

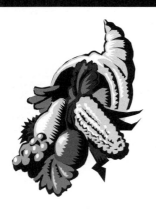

Five servings of fresh fruits and vegetables are recommended to obtain needed antioxidants.

Macular degeneration cured 35 years ago

In 1958 researchers in Helsinki believed the primary reason for macular degeneration was atherosclerosis, the progressive narrowing of the blood vessels of the retina. They identified diabetes, high blood pressure, fatigue, stress, and infections as compounding factors.

These researchers studied 71 patients 54-83 years of age, half of whom were over 70, who had both the "dry" (43) and the "wet" (19) or mixed (9) forms of macular degeneration. Some of the patients were given high doses of vitamin A and E and took heparin (a blood thinner) added to their vitamin regimen. A few only took only a vasodilator and others only a placebo (inactive pill). The vitamins were prescribed for their anti-atherosclerotic effect. More than 30,000 units of vitamin A and 70 milligrams of vitamin E were given; and the treatment varied from 4 months to 3 years. Patients were asked to draw the visual distortions they saw on paper with crossed grid lines (an Amsler grid). Retinal photographs were also taken.

Here are the results of the test:

⇒ Sixty-seven percent of the patients who took vitamin A + E and the blood thinner could see two to three more lines of letters on the eye chart than when they began the test, and many no longer had distorted vision. Only 5 percent of these patients got worse.

⇒ Of the patients who took vitamin A + E alone (without the blood thinner), 33 percent experienced two to three or more lines of visual improvement on an vision test chart. Fifteen percent of these patients got worse.

⇒ Thirty-three percent of the patients who took the vasodilator (opened up blood vessels) experienced marked improvement in their vision -- 2 or 3 or more lines of visual improvement on the eye chart. Ten percent of these patients got worse.

⇒ Patients who took inactive placebo tablets, NONE experienced any level of visual improvement and a third got worse.

The 1958 Helsinki study proved that agents which open the blood vessels (vasodilators) or that clear the blood vessels of plaques (antioxidants) resulted in improve vision

VISUAL IMPROVE-MENT	VITAMINS A +E plus a blood thinner	Vitamins A + E	Vasodilator	Placebo
MARKED VISUAL IMPROVE-MENT	67%	33%	33%	None
SLIGHT OR NO VISUAL IMPROVE-MENT	33%	67%	67%	100% None Improved

No serious complications were reported among these debilitated elderly patients. Up to the date of publication of this book, compared to this study published in 1958,[44] no other treatment has proven so effective at improving sight and preventing the progression of macular degeneration.

While the above report is noteworthy, the high doses of nutrients used are not advocated for readers of this book without consultation with a physician familiar with mega-dose nutritional therapy.

In the 1980s, German researchers essentially repeated the study performed by the Helsinki doctors in 1958 by using vitamins A and E plus a vasodilator (blood vessel widening) drug. The German doctors confirmed that such a combination of vitamins and vasodilators could actually improve vision among patients with macular degeneration.[45,46]

Now there are numerous studies that show vitamins E, C, and beta carotene (precursor for vitamin A) reduce the risk of macular degeneration.[47] Researchers found that those macular disease patients who had the highest blood levels of beta carotene, or a mixture of antioxidants (selenium, vitamin C and E), had less risk of developing macular degeneration.[48]

It appears that larger doses of antioxidant vitamins are needed to prevent macular degeneration than cataracts. The 1958 Helsinki report showed that macular disease patients experienced marked improvement in their vision when they took mega-doses of antioxidant vitamins along with a blood thinner or vasodilator. A modern study shows that normal dietary intake of antioxidants in fruits and vegetables may not afford any protection of aging retinal diseases because of their low dosage and lack of combination with blood thinners.[49]

In one study, common daily vitamin supplements from retail stores showed some anti-cataract benefit but no effect for macular degeneration.[50] Common dietary intake of antioxidants from fruits and vegetables does not appear to significantly reduce the risk of macular degeneration.[51]

Epidemiologists are reviewing large populations of adults to determine if their use of daily multi-vitamins provides any protection against macular degeneration. A number of these studies appear to indicate there is only a small benefit.[52] This is because most of these vitamin supplements provide doses of antioxidants that are sometimes less than what is consumed in the diet. For example a glass of orange juice contains as much vitamin C as most vitamin pills.

Mega-dose antioxidant formulas are advised for macular degeneration.[53] Common daily vitamin formulas offer little protection for the retina from oxidative damage. Vitamins formulas such as One-A-Day, Theragram, Centrum Silver, ZBEC, and others, while possibly adequate for younger individuals, do not provide therapeutic dosages required for retinal health. **Special antioxidant formulas should be taken by adults for macular degeneration.**

One of the primary reasons why mega-doses of nutrients have to be given to older macular degeneration patients is because they do not absorb nutrients from their foods or vitamin tablets as they once did. The lack of digestive juices impairs the ability to absorb

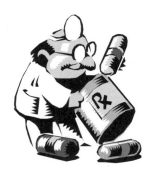

Vitamins are replacing drugs as medicines.

vitamin C, beta carotene and zinc (hydrochloric acid), vitamin E (bile), riboflavin, and most other nutrients.

The retinal light receptor cells in the center of the retina are called "cones." These cells are not readily replaced and renewed. Some researchers believe it takes up to nine months before they repair themselves. **Thus any nutritional regimen for macular degeneration should be taken for a minimum of nine months before giving up hope of visual improvement.**
Many older adults suspect that someone is trying to sell them vitamins they don't need. These suspicions should be laid aside.

Currently, nutritional therapy for macular degeneration has been confined largely to zinc supplements, plus some minimal doses of other nutrients. The current therapy has recommended far too much zinc and far to little of the other antioxidant nutrients and fatty acids that will reduce cholesterol levels.

Do zinc supplements prevent macular degeneration?

In 1988, thousands of macular disease patients made purchases at health food stores when widely circulated news reports indicated zinc may halt the progress of retinal disease.[54] Dosages of 200 milligrams were suggested and many patients began taking these mega-doses without knowledge of potential side effects, some which could exacerbate macular disease.

Compared to blue or hazel-eyed patients, it is known that brown-eyed individuals have a 20-times reduced risk of developing macular disease. The melanin colored pigment of the retina protects against sunlight-induced retinal damage. The concentration of zinc in the light receptor cells of the retina (retinal pigment epithelium) influences melanin levels. It is known that the elderly are frequently deficient in zinc, and that the aged eye begins to lose melanin pigment at age 50.[55]

The reason why a high dose of zinc was reported to be helpful for macular disease patients that commonly occurs after age 50 was probably because the zinc was helping the retard the loss of protective melanin pigment.

While zinc levels are often low in adults those who develop retinal disease often have other conditions that block the metabolism or absorption of zinc (Crohn's disease, alcoholism, pancreatitis). When zinc is deficient the macula deteriorates.[56]

It has been shown that zinc helps vitamin A to be released from the liver so that it can be used by other tissues in the body. Without zinc, vitamin A doesn't get to the retina to form rhodopsin, the chemical needed for night vision.[57,58]

While zinc is an important co-factor in the body and eyes and helps to form important antioxidant enzymes that protect the eyes from sunlight damage, too much zinc can be counter-productive. Nutritional scientists point out that zinc supplements in excess of 25 milligrams a day can rob the body of copper and also increase LDL (bad) cholesterol levels.[59] Too much zinc has been shown to create cholesterol imbalance.[60] High doses of zinc are _not_ recommended for macular degeneration. Moderate doses may be helpful when taken with other antioxidants.

Are amino acids helpful for macular degeneration?

Two amino acids, cysteine and taurine, are important for the maintenance of a healthy retina. These two amino acids are usually produced from other amino acids, but abnormal bacteria in the digestive tract can result in deficiencies and supplements may be required.

When taurine is removed from food animals develop retinal degeneration which is reversed upon the replacement of taurine[61] This amino acid is important in the maintenance of vision and the regeneration of worn out tissues of the visual system.[62]

Glutathione is a master antioxidant that protects retinal cells from light damage caused by UV and blue-violet solar radiation. Retinal cells grown in test tubes and bathed in glutathione thrive while cells without glutathione become weak.[63] Macular degeneration patients have 58 percent less glutathione than others who do not have this disease.[64,65]

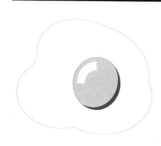

Eggs contain cysteine, an amino acid, that helps to promote the synthesis of glutathione, an important antioxidant in the body.

The production of glutathione within the body is enhanced by supplementing the diet with N-acetyl cysteine, a stable form of amino acid. Selenium and riboflavin also help to stimulate the production of glutathione.

Do fatty foods cause macular degeneration?

Humans need fat in their diet in order to survive. But too much saturated fat, which produces high cholesterol levels, too much omega-6 fats (such as from corn oil) at the expense of omega-3 fats (from cold-water fish) in the Western diet may make man more prone to develop macular degeneration.

A diet deficient in Omega-3 fats has been shown to result in visual impairment in animal eyes.[66] Omega-3 fats are so essential that when this oil is deficient in the diet the retina it begins to recycle within the eye.[67] With age, the amount of omega-3 fats decrease in the retina of animals and is believed to do the same in man.[68]

Low birth weight infants deprived of Omega-3 fats, because of feeding with cow's milk instead of breast milk, may experience visual problems. When fish oils, which contain Omega-3 fats, were added to infant formulas, visual acuities improved.[69] It appears that Omega-3 fats are both essential for nerve conduction in the retina, and to reduce cholesterol, thus helping to maintain retinal nutrition by keeping retinal blood vessels open.

While Omega-3 fats are beneficial to the cardiovascular and ocular systems, there is one drawback with these fats. Any fats exposed to sunlight spoil or turn rancid, a process called lipid peroxidation. The more Omega-3 fats in the diet, the more antioxidant protection from vitamins C, E and beta carotene is required.[70] Lipid peroxidation (spoilage of fat) is believed to be involved in retinal degenerations.[71]

Over a four-week period, when European researchers gave infusions of Omega-3 fats to seven patients over age 70 who had macular degeneration, six of the seven patients experienced a subjective improvement in vision.[72]

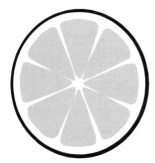

Bioflavonoids are pigments found in the skin of plants that protect from sunlight damage. Quercetin, a bioflavonoid found in red onions, has similar properties to melanin, the natural pigment at the back of the eyes.

Are bioflavonoids helpful for macular degeneration?

Bioflavonoids are plant pigments that have special health promoting properties, especially for the eyes. Bioflavonoids are found in red onions, cherries, red grapes, huckleberries and citrus fruits; more than 4000 plants contain bioflavonoids. Plants use bioflavonoids for protection from sunlight damage. A particular type of bioflavonoid (anthocyanidins) absorb sunlight similar to melanin in the retina of the eye.[73]

When 31 patients with retinal disorders, including diabetic retinopathy, were given bioflavonoids (anthocyanosides) less hemorrhage was noted.[74]

When 10 macular degeneration patients (average age 67 years) were given 80 milligrams of bioflavonoids twice daily (160 milligrams total of ginko biloba), distance vision improved in nine of these patients over a sixth month period; none deteriorated. The vision of only two patients taking a placebo tablet improved while four deteriorated.[75]

Bioflavonoids such as rutin (derived from buckwheat), have been used to reduce the leakage from small blood vessels (capillaries) in the retina.[76] This may be important to diabetics and older adults who have the "wet" or leaky form of macular degeneration.

Quercetin, a bioflavonoid that contains anthocyanosides, has been shown to be the most potent of all the bioflavonoids in reducing the spoilage (lipid peroxidation) of fats in eye tissues caused by ultraviolet light.[77] The attack by sun rays upon the polyunsaturated fats that comprise the membranes of retinal cells is believed to be a primary cause of their degeneration. Antioxidants such as bioflavonoids, and cell-wall stabilizer taurine, and vitamin E may help protect the retina from deterioration.[78]

Does coffee worsen macular degeneration?

Caffeine is available in a wide variety of beverages and foods. Approximately 20-30 percent of the general population ingests more than 500-600 milligrams of this drug daily, equivalent to 2-3 cups of coffee. **Researchers have now shown that there is a 13**

percent reduction in retinal blood flow after caffeine intake. Caffeine also appears to increase blood pressure and may cause the blood vessels to constrict to some degree. The effect of caffeine upon the retinal circulation may be of importance to older adults whose retinal blood vessels have already narrowed due to atherosclerosis, blood clots, calcification, or vasospasm.[79]

Is aspirin helpful for macular degeneration?

Aspirin, by virtue of the fact it thins the blood and increases blood flow to the retina, has been recommended as a therapeutic treatment for macular degeneration.

Physicians frequently prescribe aspirin to treat blood vessel diseases and to prevent temporary blockages of oxygen to the brain, a condition called transient ischemic attack. The use of aspirin to improve blood flow to the retina has been recommended.[80] In one human study it was shown that aspirin decreases the risk of macular degeneration by 20 percent.[81]

Patients taking as little as 75 milligrams of aspirin have been shown to develop hemorrhages in their retina. The same is true for pain relievers like iboprofen.[82] In another report, a patient taking 650 milligrams of aspirin developed hemorrhages.[83] Macular degeneration patients may be at an increased risk to develop retinal bleeding, especially if they have high blood pressure. Non-steroidal anti-inflammatory pain pills can also cause similar problems. While aspirin may be an effective way of preventing the blood platelets to form into clots within the body, there may be some side effects.[84]

Aspirin use by macular degeneration patients is not recommended and should be discouraged. Seek consultation with an eye physician.

Caffeine reduces retinal blood flow by 13 percent.

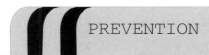

NUTRITION

PREVENTION

Summary of preventive measures

The importance of keeping the retinal blood vessels open cannot be overemphasized. These tiny blood capillaries can narrow due to the buildup of cholesterol, blood clots (called thrombi) and calcifications, or they can close up and spasm. Narrowing of the carotid artery is an additional factor.

The result of these vascular occlusive retinal disorders is that the retina becomes starved of antioxidants carried in the blood stream to protect the retina from sunlight damage. When these blood vessels become severely closed, the retina is starved for oxygen and new abnormal blood vessels, the "wet" form of macular degeneration, begin to grow. While older individuals may begin with the "dry" form of macular disease, if their retinal arteries become occluded they could also develop the more serious "wet" form of the disease.

People who develop macular degeneration can be identified by their eye doctors years before vision is lost. These high risk patients are blue eyed, have lots of solar aging spots on their retinas (drusen), and may have a family history of the disease. These patients should be advised to take preventive measures for the remainder of their lives. **Patients should ask their eye physicians if they have the drusen aging spots at the back of their eyes; about 30 percent of adults do.**

By the year 2020, an estimated 7.5 million American adults will suffer with vision loss caused by macular degeneration. Adults who were born during the years 1940 to 1955 will comprise the age group of older Americans who will be age 65 to 80 beginning in the year 2020. If our

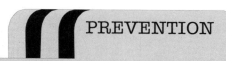

society is to avert a visual and economic disaster, this population, the "baby boomers," need to practice preventive measures beginning immediately is to avert a visual and economic disaster.

The medical literature reveals that macular degeneration cannot only be stopped in its tracks but reversed in some cases. This eye disease is not without hope. The purpose of this book, however, is not to give macular degeneration patients false hopes; those who have promoted Interferon injections have already made that mistake.

If beginning a nutritional regimen, **have the persistence to continue taking supplements for at least nine to twelve months.** The cells at the back of the eyes may take that long to regenerate.

The following is a simple regimen for macular degeneration patients to follow:

• Take 1000 milligrams of vitamin C daily. Start with smaller doses and work up to 1000 milligrams to avoid diarrhea.

• Take 20,000-40,000 units of vitamin A activity from beta carotene daily.

• Take 400-800 units of vitamin E daily.

• Take 500-1000 mg. of omega-3 oils a day to reduce cholesterol deposits and blood clots in small blood vessels of the eyes.

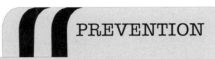

NUTRITION

PREVENTION

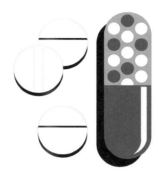

Capsules absorb better than tablets

• Dosages of omega-3 fatty acids can be taken in stronger dosages (1500-2500 mgs.) for a short period of time (2 weeks). Then the dosage should be reduced to 1000 mg. daily.

• Take 1000 milligrams of garlic in capsules to prevent blood clots (thrombi) from forming in the small blood vessels of the retina and to reduce cholesterol.

• Take 100 milligrams of N-acetyl cysteine (a glutathione precursor) daily.

• Take 15-25 milligrams of zinc daily.

• Take 100 micrograms of selenium daily.

• Take 100 milligrams of the amino acid taurine daily.

• Take 1000-3000 milligrams of bioflavonoids derived from quercetin, bilberry or ginko biloba capsules. Quercetin + Vitamin C by Nature's Herbs is an excellent product. Start with low doses and work up to optimal doses to avoid diarrhea.

The dosages of vitamins outlined above can be found in health food stores. Become familiar with brand names and learn how to read labels for dosages and number of ingredients. Pills in capsule form are more easily absorbed then hard tablets.

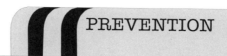

NUTRITION   PREVENTION

In this author's own research the following formulas have been found to contain the correct ratio and quantity of ingredients. These formulas below should also eliminate the need to take 20 pills a day.

⇒ Take 2 capsules of Maxilife CoQ10 formula by Twinlab daily.

⇒ Take 2 capsules of Ocuguard by Twinlab daily.

⇒ Take 1000 milligrams of garlic capsules daily. The enteric-coated garlic capsules by Nature's Herbs minimize garlic breath.

⇒ Various brands of omega-3 oils are available at local health food stores. Take 1000 milligrams of omega-3 oils from flax seed daily until improvement is noticed. Then 500 milligrams thereafter for health maintenance.

⇒ Wear 100 percent UV-blue violet filtering wrap-around sun lenses.

⇒ The diet should be very low in saturated fats, preferably 10 percent of calories should come from saturated fats. This means avoidance of meats and dairy products.

⇒ Smokers should enroll in a smoking cessation program.

⇒ Limit caffeine intake from coffee, sodas, tea.

⇒ Avoid aspirin and ibuprofen even in low doses.

Preventive therapy should begin when early signs of the disease, such as aging spots (drusen) at the back of the eyes are observed. These spots can be observed early in life.

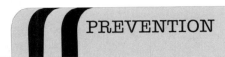

NUTRITION

PREVENTION

This regimen of prevention is no guarantee one will get any of their vision back or even prevent further vision loss. Many ophthalmologists observe that their patients' vision improves or is preserved when taking these formulas. Certainly patients have improved with a combination of antioxidants rather than with zinc alone.

Macular disease patients should be armed with an Amsler Grid home vision test which they take every day. In this way they can call their eye doctor at the first sign of progressive vision loss. The Amsler grid test should be taken on vacations or whenever away from home.

Macular disease patients should make their family members aware that they are at an increased risk of developing macular degeneration during their lifetime.

Macular degeneration IS preventable and in some cases reversible. Read the section in this book series on circulatory eye problems.

Vision Test

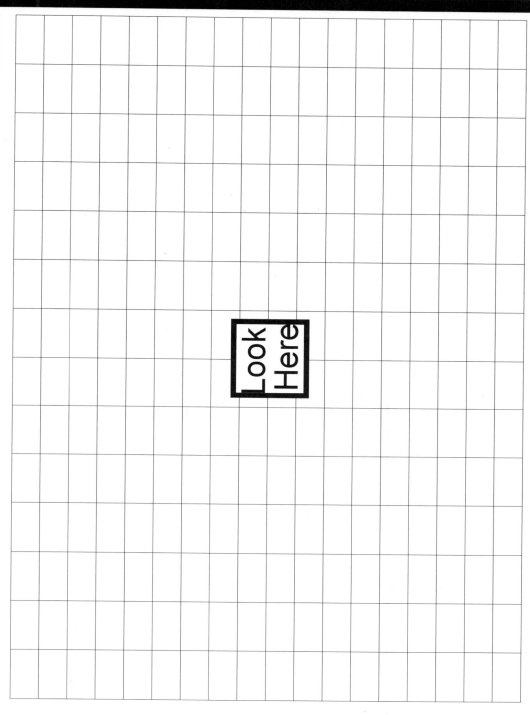

Home Vision Test
1. **Turn this page sideways.**
2. **Use with reading light. Hold at reading distance.**
3. **Cover one eye.**
4. **Look at the center dot and keep your eyes on the center at all times.**
5. **Note wavy, fuzzy areas.**
6. **Test your other eye. If abnormalities are observed or have become bigger, contact an eye physician.**

REFERENCES

[1] Albert D.M. and F.A. Jacobiec, PRINCIPLES OF OPHTHALMOLOGY, W. B. Saunders Co., Philadelphia, 1994.

[2] Smith-Brewer S., "Vision loss in age-related maculopathy: primary care referral guide," Geriatrics 42: 99-106, 1987.

[3] Ferris F.L., "Senile macular degeneration: review of epidemiologic features," American Journal of Epidemiology 118: 132-50, 1983.

[4] Roy M., Kaiser-Kupfer M., "Second eye involvement in age-related macular degeneration: a four year prospective study," Investigative Ophthalmology, 31: ARVO Abstracts, March 15, 1990.

[5] Witzleben J.C., "Physician-artist describes own experience with macular disease," Ophthalmology Times, March 1984, p. 1 & 32.

[6] Alexander M.F., et al, "Assessment of visual function in patients with age-related macular degeneration and low visual acuity," Archives of Ophthalmology 106: 1543-47, 1988.

[7] Ferris F.L., "Age-related macular degeneration and blindness due to neovascular maculopathy," Archives of Ophthalmology 102: 1640-42, 1984.

[8] Stangler-Zuschrott E., "Reduced reading speed and early fatigue as indicators of impaired vision," Klin Mbl. Augenheilk, 196: 150-57, 1990.

[9] Steinmetz R.L., Walker D., Fitzke F.W., Bird A.C., "Prolonged dark adaptation in patients with age related macular degeneration," Investigative Ophthalmology, 32: ARVO Abstracts, March 15, 1991.

[10] Peterson S., "Macular degeneration relieved by interferon, doctor reports," Orange County Register, October 16, 1991, p. A16.

[11] Polinar L.S., Tournambe P.E., "Interferon alpha 2A for subfoveal neovascularization in age-related macular degeneration," Investigative Ophthalmology, 34: 2246-10, March 15, 1993.

[12] Thomas M.A., Ibanez H.E., "Interferon Alfa-2a in the treatment of subfoveal choroidal neovascularization," American Journal of Ophthalmology 115: 563-68, 1993.

[13]

[14] Yannuzzi, L.A., "A new standard of care for laser photocoagulation for subfoveal choroidal neovascularization secondary to age-related macular degeneration," Archives of Ophthalmology 112: 480-88, 1994.

[15] Eldred K.B., "Optimal illumination for reading in patients with age-related maculopathy," Optometry and Vision Sciences 69: 46-50, 1992.

[16] Gawande A., Marmor M.F., "The specificity of colored lenses in aiding visual performance in retinal disease," Report, Stanford University Medical Center, 1991.

[17] Virtanen P., Laatikainen L.,"Acta Ophthalmologica 69: 484-90, 1991.

[18] Eldred K.B., "Optimal illumination for reading in patients with age-related maculopathy," Optometry & Vision Science, 69: 46-50, 1992.

[19] "Mini-TV screens in wraparound sunglasses," NASA Report, July 1988.

[20] Elliott D.B., Whitaker D., "Changes in macular function throughout adulthood," Documenta Ophthalmologica 76: 251-59, 1991.

[21] Vinding T., Appleyard M., Nyboe J., Jensen G., "Risk factor analysis for atrophic and exudative age-related macular degeneration," Acta Ophthalmologica 70: 66-72, 1992.

[22] Paetkau M.E., et al, "Senile disciform macular degeneration and smoking," Canadian Journal of Ophthalmology 13: 67-71, 1978.

[23] Organisciak D.T., Wang H., Yi-Li Z., Tso M.O.M., "The protective effect of ascorbate in retinal light damage of rats," Ophthalmology & Visual Sciences, 26: 1580-88, 1985.

[24] Organisciak D.T., Jiang Y., Wang H., Bicknell I., "The protective effect of ascorbic acid in retinal light damage of rats exposed to intermittent light," Investigative Ophthalmology & Visual Science, 31: 1195-1202, 1990.

[25] Blumenkranz M.S., et al, "Risk factors in age-related maculopathy complicated by choroidal neovascularization," Ophthalmology 93: 552-58, 1986.

[26] van de Hoeve J., "Eye lesions produced by light rich in ultraviolet rays: senile cataract, senile degeneration of the macula," American Journal of Ophthalmology 3: 178-94, 1920.

[27] Drucker B.L., Shapiro L.A., "Protective effect of occlusion on disciform degeneration," Annals of Ophthalmology 20: 118-19, 1988.

[28] Munoz B., et al, "Blue light and risk of age-related macular degeneration," Investigative Ophthalmology 31: ARVO Abstracts, March 15, 1990.

[29] Cruickshanks K.J., Klein R., Klein B.E.K., "Sunlight and age-related macular degneration," Archives of Ophthalmology 111: 514-18, 1993.

[30] Smith H.E., "Actinic macular retinal pigment degeneration," U.S. Naval Medical Bulletin 42: 675-80, 1944.

[31] Chumbley L.C., "Impressions of eye diseases among Rhodesian blacks in Moshonaland," South African Medical Journal 52: 316-18, 1977.

[32] Smith S.C, Dhindsa H.S., Rapp L.M., "Photoreceptor cell damage and renewal following exposure to ultraviolet-A light," Experimental Eye Research 32: ARVO Abstracts, March 15, 1991.

[33] Werner J.S., Steele V.G., Pfoff D.S., "Loss of human photoreceptor sensitivity associated with chronic exposure to ultraviolet radiation," Ophthalmology 96: 1552-58, 1989.

[34] Goldman A.I., Ham W.T., Mueller H.A., "Ocular damage thresholds and mechanisms for ultrashort pulses of both visible and infrared laser radiation in the rhesus monkey," Experimental Eye Research 24: 45-56, 1977.

[35] West S.K., eet al, "Exposure to sunlight and other risk factors for age-related macular degeneration," Archives of Ophthalmology 107: 875-79, 1989.

[36] Liu I.Y., White L., LaCroix A.Z., "The association of age-related macular degeneration and lens opacities in the aged," American Journal of Public Health 79: 765-69, 1989.

[37] Mainster M., "Light and macular degeneration: a biophysical and clinical prespective," Eye 1: 304-10, 1987.

[38] van Kujik F., "Effects of ultraviolet light on the eye: role of protective glasses," Environmental Health Perspectives 96: 177-84, 1991.

[39] Young R.W., "Solar radiation and age-related macular degeneration," Survey of Ophthalmology 32: 252-69, 1988.

[40] Sternberg P., "Treating age-related macular degeneration," Research to Prevent Blindness Science Writers Seminar, 1992.

[41] Hoover D.L., Robb R.M., Peterson R.A., "Optic disc drusen in children," Journal of Pediatric Ophthalmology & Strabismus, 25: 191-95, 1988.

[42] Rosenthal F.S., et al, "The effect of sunglasses on ocular exposure to ultraviolet radiation," American Journal of Public Health, 78: 72-74, 1988.

[43] Handelman G.J., Dratz E.A., "The role of antioxidants in the retina and retinal pigment epithelium and the nature of prooxidant-induced damage," Advances in Free Radical Biology & Medicine, 2: 1-89, 1986.

[44] Vannas S., Orma H., "On the treatment of arteriosclerotic chorioretinopathy," Acta Ophthalmologica 36: 601-12, 1958.

[45] Stark H., "Long-term treatment of senilr degeneration of the macula with Cosaldon A + E," Klin. Mbl. Augenheilk, 187: 296-302, 1985.

[46] Flamm P., "Treatment of degenerative maculopathy with Cosaldon A + E," Klin. Mbl. Augenheilk, 190: 59-66, 1987.

[47] Hyman L., et al, "Risk factors for age-related maculopathy," Investigative Ophthalmology, 33: ARVO Abstracts 548, March 15, 1992.

[48] Eye Disease Case Control Study Group, "Antioxidant status and neovascular age-related macular degeneration," Archives of Ophthalmology 111: 104-09, 1993.

[49] Drews C.D., et al, "Dietary antioxidants and age related macular degeneration," Investigative Ophthalmology 34: ARVO Abstracts 2237-1, March 15, 1993.

[50] Vitale S., et al, "Vitamin supplement use, age related macular degeneration, and cataract in Chesapeake Bay Watermen, Investigative Ophthalmology, 34: ARVO Abstracts 1785, March 15, 1993.

[51] Drews C.D., et al, Dietary antioxidants and age related macular degeneration," Investigative Ophthalmology, 34: ARVO Abstracts 2237, March, 15, 1993

[52] Mares-Perlman J.A., et al, "Relationships between age-related maculopathy and intake of vitamin and mineral supplements," Investigative Ophthalmology 34: ARVO Abstracts 2121, March 15, 1993.

[53] Pizzorno J., Murray M., ENCYCLOPEDIA OF NATURAL MEDICINE, Prima, 1990.

[54] Kolata G., "Zinc shows promise in slowing disease that causes blindness," The New York Times, March 10, 1988.

[55] Weiter, J.J., et al, "Relationship of senile macular degeneration to ocular pigmentation," American Journal of Ophthalmology 99: 185-87, 1985.

[56] Tso M.O.M., RETINAL DISEASES, J.B. Lippincott, Philadelphia, 1988, p. 289.

[57] Wong E.K., "Leopold I.H., "Zinc deficiency and visual dysfunction," Metabolic Pediatric Ophthalmology 3: 1-4, 1979.

[58] Shuster T., Conly D., "Light enhanced binding of zinc to rhodopsin," Investigative Ophthalmology, 31: ARVO Abstracts, March 15, 1990.

[59] McClain C.J., Stuart M.A., "Zinc metabolism in the elderly," in GERIATRIC NUTRITION, John E. Morley, editor, Raven Press, New York, 1990.

[60] Haausmann P., THE RIGHT DOSE, Ballantine, New York, 1987.

[61] Rapp L.M., "Synergism between environmental lighting and taurine depletion in causing photoreceptor cell degeneration," Experimental Eye Research 46: 229-38, 1988.

[62] Anyanwu E., "The neurochemical involvement of taurine in ocular pathology," Metabolic, Pediatric and Systemic Ophthalmology 15: 21-24, 1992.

[63] Sternberg P., "Treating age-related macular degeneration," Science Writers Seminar in Ophthalmology, Research to Prevent Blindness, 1988.

[64] Sternberg P., "Protection of retinal pigment epithelium from oxidative injury by glutathione and precursors," Investigative Ophthalmology 34: 3661-68, 1993.

[65] Prashar S., et al, "Antioxidant enzymes in RBC's as a biological index of age related macular degeneration," Acta Ophthalmologica 71: 214-18, 1993.

[66] Connor W.E., Neuringer M., Reisbick S., "Essential fatty acids: the important of n-3 fatty acids in the retina and brain," Nutrition Reviews 50: 21-29, 1992.

[67] Stinson A.M., Wiegand R.D., Anderson R.E., "Recycling of docosohexaenoic acid in rat retinas during n-3 fatty acid deficiency," Journal of Lipid Research 32: 2009-17, 1991.

Ophthalmology, Research to Prevent Blindness, 1988.

[64] Sternberg P., "Protection of retinal pigment epithelium from oxidative injury by glutathione and precursors," Investigative Ophthalmology 34: 3661-68, 1993.

[65] Prashar S., et al, "Antioxidant enzymes in RBC's as a biological index of age related macular degeneration," Acta Ophthalmologica 71: 214-18, 1993.

[66] Connor W.E., Neuringer M., Reisbick S., "Essential fatty acids: the important of n-3 fatty acids in the retina and brain," Nutrition Reviews 50: 21-29, 1992.

[67] Stinson A.M., Wiegand R.D., Anderson R.E., "Recycling of docosohexaenoic acid in rat retinas during n-3 fatty acid deficiency," Journal of Lipid Research 32: 2009-17, 1991.

[68] "Age decreases the n-3 polyunsaturated fatty acids of the retina," Nutrition Reviews 47: 87-89, 1989.

[69] Birch E.E., et al, Investigative Ophthalmology 33: 3242-53, 1992.

[70] Bush R.A., Reme C.E., Malnoe A., "Light damage in the rat retina: the effect of dietary deprivation of N-3 fatty acids on acute structural alterations," Experimental Eye Research 53: 741-52, 1991.

[71] Anderson R.E., Rapp L.M., Wiegand R.D., "Lipid peroxidation and retinal degeneration," Current Eye Research 3: 223-27, 1984.

[72] Heidrich H., Harnisch J.P., Ranft J., "PGE1 in senile macular degeneration: a pilot study," Klin Mbl. Augenheilk. 194: 282-84, 1989.

[73] Leibovitz B., "Catechins and anthocyanidins: potent polyphenols," Manuscript, December 3, 1992.

[74] Scharrer A., Ober M., "Anthocyanosides in the treatment of retinopathies," Klin. Mbl. Augenehilk. 178: 386-89, 1981.

[75] Lebuisson D.A., Leroy L., Rigal G., "Treatment of senile macular degeneration with ginko biloba extract," in ROKAN (GINKO BILOBA) RECENT RESULTS IN PHARMACOLOGY AND CLINIC, E.W. Funfgeld, editor, Springer-Verlag, New York, 1988, pp. 231-36.

[76] Somerville-Large L.B., "A note on the clinical value of rutin in ophthalmology," Transactions Ophthalmological Society United Kingdom, 69: 615-17, 1950.

[77] Devamanoharan P.S., Varma S., "Anti-lipid peroxidative efficacy of flavonoids in ocular tissues," Investigative Ophthalmology, 31: ARVO Abstracts, March 15, 1990.

[78] Hunyor A.B.L., "Solar retinopathy: its significance for the ageing eye and the younger pseudophakic patient," Australian and New Zealand Journal of Ophthalmology 15: 371-75, 1987.

[79] Lotti K, Grunwald J.E., "The effect of caffeine on the human macular circulation," Investigative Ophthalmology 32: 3028-32, 1991.

[80] Kana J.S., "Effect of long-term aspirin therapy on ophthalmic artery blood flow in patients with carotid atherosclerotic disease," Investigative Ophthalmology, 34: ARVO Abstracts 3410, March 15, 1993.

[81] Christen W.G., et al, "Aspirin and age-related maculopathy," Investigative Ophthalmology 34: 2120,

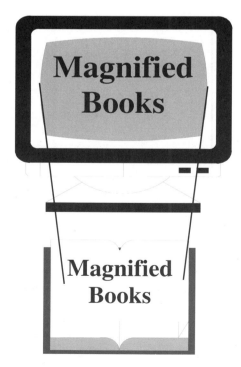

Various computer devices are available to magnify printed materials for the visually impaired. Check with your eye physician or low vision center.

Quick facts

<u>Part of the eye affected</u>-- peripheral retina, lens

<u>Typical age of onset</u>-- night vision problems in youth

<u>Risk factors</u>-- family history, drug interactions

<u>Modern treatment</u>-- none

<u>Preventive measures</u>-- antioxidant nutritional supplements, UV-blocking sunglasses

<u>Questions to ask your eye doctor:</u>

Will diet help control this disorder? Can special sunglasses help RP patients? How often do I need to obtain eye examinations?

3
RETINITIS PIGMENTOSA

Don is in his forties and was diagnosed with retinitis pigmentosa years ago. His vision is fine so far and his ophthalmologist has suggested he take antioxidant supplements to help maintain his sight or at least to slow down the eventual progression of visual loss. After taking the nutritional supplements for over a year he suddenly notices that his skin is turning yellow. He develops what is called a beta carotene tan. Don takes so much beta carotene that all of it cannot be stored in his liver in the form of vitamin A. Some is being stored in his skin. Oftentimes a beta carotene tan is mistaken for a case of jaundice. But Don's eyes are white. He doesn't have jaundice. Reducing the dosage of beta carotene will resolve Don's problem.

Under further questioning Don indicates his blood cholesterol level is unusually low. Recently he has also experienced considerable air and gas following meals. He admits he has a habit of swallowing food quickly. These are signs that Don isn't producing the digestive juices required to absorb nutrients, especially fats, from his diet or the vitamin capsules.

Beta carotene requires a small amount of fat to convert into vitamin A. Don's low cholesterol level may indicate he has a fat absorption problem. Abnormally low levels of vitamin A are known to result in poor night vision, the foremost sign of retinitis pigmentosa. Don is advised to see his physician and to consider taking digestive enzymes that contain bile, pancreatin, pepsin and hydrochloric acid to improve absorption of nutrients. Don's story suggests that there may be metabolic disorders outside of the eyes that may be linked to retinitis pigmentosa.

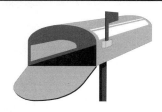

Mail bag

I wondered if you could tell me anything about retinitis pigmentosa. This disease runs in my family. I have three nephews in 35-40 range with it and a sister now 65 showing signs of it. Would appreciate any help you can provide.

H.R.
Lincoln, Nebraska

What is retinitis pigmentosa?

Retinitis pigmentosa refers to a family of eye disorders where pigment clumps at the back of the eyes in the retina causing night blindness. The result here is slow progressive loss of side vision leading to tunnel vision and eventual blindness. Visual problems often begin in childhood but don't produce severe visual symptoms until later in life. The family of RP eye diseases includes Refsum's Disease, Usher's Disease, Sturge-Webber syndrome, gyrate atrophy, Leber's Hereditary Dystrophy as well as other varieties such as X-linked and simplex. There are 14 different types of primary retinitis pigmentosa.

What are the common misconceptions about RP?

John R. Heckenlively M.D. of the Jules Stein Eye Institute, lists the common myths about RP.[1]

It is untrue that nothing can be done about RP. In at least one form of RP (abetalipoproteinemia), which may occur as early as age two, vitamin A supplements can improve adaptation to night vision.[2] There are other measures that can be prescribed for each variety of retinitis pigmentosa.

Contrary to what you may have heard, most RP patients do not become deaf. Actually deafness accompanies Usher's Syndrome, one of the family of retinitis pigmentosa disorders. This syndrome should not be confused with adult onset deafness. Only 6-10 percent of RP patients have Usher's variety of RP.

RP patients do not suddenly go blind. RP progresses slowly.

All RP patients do not become night blind during childhood. Many retinitis pigmentosa patients don't notice night vision problems till later in life.

Contrary to popular belief retinitis pigmentosa is not inherited from the mother. Actually only one-third to one-half of RP patients have a genetically-based retinal disorder.[3]

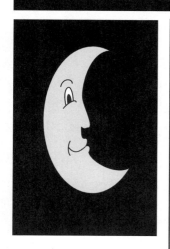

Night vision problems are the hallmark sign of retinitis pigmentosa.

The cause of retinitis pigmentosa is not pigment which gets in the way of the light. Actually light receptor cells are being destroyed.

How many have RP?

The worldwide prevalence of retinitis pigmentosa is one in 4000 to one in 7500 persons. A family history of RP suggests genetic counseling and continued eye examinations throughout life.

How do retinitis pigmentosa patients cope with their visual problems?

The typical retinitis pigmentosa patient complains of night blindness dating from their childhood years, with noticeable loss of side vision in their late twenties. Youngsters with RP often are seen as clumsy and awkward, running into things which people with normal sight can see. In their forties RP patients experience narrowed vision and severe night blindness; nearly half will develop cataracts. Other visual problems are also common, such as focusing problems, reading vision difficulty, light sensitivity, and headaches.

Because of difficulties with night vision, most RP patients restrict driving to daylight hours. Use of additional mirrors and turning the head make up for some loss of side vision.

Most RP patients are quite dependent upon sunglasses during the day. A small group of RP patients indicate their vision improves with red lenses.[4]

Retinitis pigmentosa patients frequently experience depression, anxiety, and anger against relatives, their physician, or even God for having allowed this disease to happen. Most RP patients have some useful vision throughout the first half of their life. The impending threat of severe visual loss may cause greater anxiety than the sudden loss of sight. Most RP patients are not motivated to use braille but with time will use magnifiers.

When questioned, not all RP patients complain of night vision problems. Some eye doctors place two or three silver coins on the floor of a dimly lighted exam room to see if RP children can find them.[5]

What is the treatment for RP?

There is no surgical, laser or medical approach to RP. Treatment is confined to cataract extraction when lens opacities occur, prescription magnifiers, low vision aids, and other preventive measures.

In 1991, Italian researchers reported on the use of a ganglioside-derived drug (GM1, Sygen, Fidia Pharmaceutical). Researchers used this drug with 40 RP patients on 73 eyes that could be tested and determined that it improved the peripheral vision in 18 of these eyes and stabilized the vision of 43 eyes. In 18 of 80 eyes visual acuity actually improved. This was a preliminary study but it does give hope with further investigation that there will be new "cures" for RP.[6]

The genetic marker for retinitis pigmentosa was discovered in 1989 on chromosome 3, but it is not known how this discovery will help to prevent or treat RP patients. Prenatal testing could help to identify individuals who are at risk to develop the disease.[7] More recently, a variety of RP in animals was prevented by injecting an artificial gene into fertilized eggs.[8]

In 1988, researchers were able to grow retinal pigmented epithelial cells. In retinitis pigmentosa, pigmented epithelial cells are abnormal and the waste products shed from them clump instead of being carried away. These home-grown healthy pigmented epithelial cells were injected into animal eyes and repeatedly reversed the disease. There is hope that this approach may some day renew sight for those individuals who are already afflicted with RP.[9]

Night vision goggles have been tried and found useful among RP patients, though they are used only experimentally at the present time.[10]

Can RP be prevented?

What causes the pigment at the back of the eyes to clump up and rob individuals of their sight? If doctors knew this they might be able to conquer this serious eye disorder. Despite many years of investigation and million of dollars of research, the cause of RP has escaped identification. Here's what researchers do know about RP.

Is RP caused by drug side effects?

Photosensitizing drugs, medications that react to UV sun rays, can sometimes cause retinal pigment cells to clump and can worsen or induce retinal disorders. The most common of these sun-sensitive drugs are chloroquine, stelazine, Mellaril, thiazide tranquilizers, tetracycline, sulfa and diuretics.[11] These drugs should be avoided by RP patients and those with a history of RP in their family. Given that only one-third to one-half of the cases of RP are genetically based, and that certain sun-sensitive drugs can mimic symptoms of RP,[12] medical detectives should further explore the possibility that the side effects of these drugs may cause many cases of this irreversible family of eye diseases. RP patients who have "bulls eye" defects in their retinas are the most likely suspects for drug-induced RP.

An interesting report shows that in an extended family of 54 individuals with a history of RP, 29 percent exhibited a prevalence of a condition called bull's eye maculopathy and a 14 percent prevalence of optic nerve drusen; much higher than would be expected for a group of unrelated patients.[13]

Bull's eye maculopathy is a condition where a doughnut-shaped hole in the retinal pigment epithelium appears. This doughnut hole in the retina appears where there is an accumulation of aging spots (lipofuscin) in the retina. The center of the retina (macula) is filled with melanin that protects the retina from sunlight damage. Photosensitizing medications bind to the melanin and leave the retina prone to light damage.[14]

In suspected cases of optic nerve disease secondary to medications Irving H. Leopold M.D. suggests patients take supplements of zinc, 1000 mcgs. of vitamin B12 and 300 mg. of thiamine.[15]

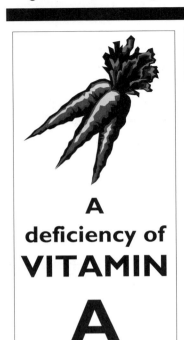

A deficiency of **VITAMIN A** results in night vision problems

Sunlight and RP

Retinitis pigmentosa patients who work outdoors have a more severe form of RP than those who work indoors. The light receptor cells at the back of the eyes that are used for night vision are called rods. Rod cells can be damaged by UV and blue-violet sun rays, and bleaching of the chemicals used for night vision by exposure to intense sun rays during the day results in diminished night vision. To maximize the retinal chemicals for night vision, wear UV and blue-violet protective sun lenses outdoors during daylight hours.

Fatty acids and RP

The rod cells renew themselves every two weeks. In at least one form of retinitis pigmentosa a lack of fatty acids (oils) from the diet resulted in disorganized cell renewal.[16] Omega-3 and Omega-6 oils are essential in the diet. In another study, 73 percent of male RP patients over age 35 had high cholesterol levels, compared to 27 percent among non-RP subjects.[17] Saturated fat intake appears to exacerbate RP.

Vitamin A and RP

There has been a continued interest in the role of vitamin A in retinitis pigmentosa. This is because a deficiency of vitamin A results in night vision problems; rod cells (night vision cells) die when deprived of vitamin A and sunlight damages retinal cells more easily when vitamin A levels are low.[18]

Various attempts have been made to find a cure for RP using vitamin A, amino acids, vasodilators, placental tissue, yeast and a variety of other approaches.

A variety of the oxidation process, called singlet oxygen, has been identified as the agent that destroys night vision cells in the retinas of RP patients. Nature's most efficient protectant from singlet oxygen is beta carotene, a natural plant pigment that is obtained from the diet and turns to vitamin A in the liver.

Pigmentary retinal problems have been reported to occur when liver or digestive tract problems occur.[19] A small amount of fat is required for efficient absorption of beta carotene, as well as vitamin A from the gut. Thyroid disorders may also affect vitamin A levels. When the bile duct is cut, pigmentary degeneration of the retina also results.[20]

Patients with liver disease or chronic pancreatitis develop night blindness. When these patients are treated with vitamin A alone no improvement is noticed. But when zinc is combined with vitamin A, improvement is noted. Chronic alcoholics are often both zinc and vitamin A deficient.[21] Zinc helps vitamin A to be released from the liver.

It is also interesting to note that RP patients typically have low zinc levels, and that zinc deficiency is often seen in cases of liver disease and pancreatitis.[22]

The reason why vitamin A supplements are recommended rather than beta carotene is that vitamin A is five times easier to absorb.[23] However, if beta carotene is taken with meals which usually have some fat content, absorption increases.

Researchers recently gained public attention when they reported that relatively high doses of vitamin A (15,000 units of vitamin A palmitate) may slow down the progress of RP. This study did not show an improvement in vision, just a slowing of the deterioration measured by the electrical energy output of the retina. According to calculations in this study, the average RP patient who would go blind at age 63 could still experience sight up till age 70 if they supplemented their diet with vitamin A supplements. When high dose vitamin E (400 units) was combined with vitamin A the preventive effect was reduced.[24] [Author's note: Vitamin E is essential. Take vitamin E supplements at different times of the day than vitamin A to maximize absorption.] Oddly, a similar group of RP patients who did not take vitamin supplements exhibited half the rate of visual decline compared to this study.[25] So the value of this study, the advice to take vitamin A instead of beta carotene, and to stop vitamin E, must be evaluated carefully.

In 1978, researchers discovered that if the vitamin therapy begins prior to age 30 large daily doses of vitamin A can have a dramatic effect on the preservation of side vision among RP patients.[26]

Link between skin and retinal disorders?

There is a linkage between skin disorders and at least some forms of retinitis pigmentosa. A skin condition known as Darier's disease is sometimes accompanied by retinitis pigmentosa. Patients with this disorder exhibit brittle nails, a sign of fatty acid deficiency or malabsorption. Vitamin B6 and fatty acid supplements (omega-6 fats in evening primrose oil) may be helpful for both of these conditions.[27] This study attempted to emphasize that the poor metabolism of vitamin A, rather than a deficiency, may be the root of the skin and eye problems.[28]

A diet low in fat and high in carbohydrates was shown to significantly slow the progress of RP in animal eyes.[29]

Taurine and RP

The amino acid taurine, 1000 mg., when taken with vitamin E, 800 mg., in half doses twice a day, improved vision among those with the autosomal dominant form of RP and those with Usher's syndrome. (The simplex and recessive forms of RP meanwhile remained stable, and the X-linked group showed no stabilization or improvement.)[30]

Researchers showed a relationship between taurine deficiency and progression of retinal degeneration. Taurine deficient animal retinas, when exposed to light, degenerated.[31] No one can ignore the fact that light and nutrition play an important role in RP and that taurine levels combine both of these factors.

Vitamin E and retinitis pigmentosa

The role of vitamin E in retinitis pigmentosa is of interest. Patients with a deficiency of vitamin A and E are known to develop night blindness and retinal degeneration; similar to RP.[32] One patient who developed a pigmentary retinal disease was found to have a malabsorption problem for vitamin E. It took more than eight years before the vision of this patient was affected.[33] Vitamin E is a fatty vitamin and is so essential to the human body that it is stored in the liver and can be called up when needed.

Digestion and RP

Without bile secreted by the liver, fatty vitamins like vitamin A and E cannot be adequately absorbed and utilized.[34] Patients who experience night blindness have been shown to have low levels of vitamin A and E from malabsorption problems.[35]

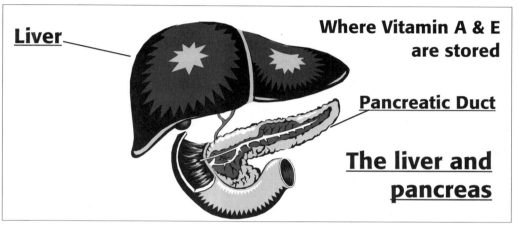

Liver

Where Vitamin A & E are stored

Pancreatic Duct

The liver and pancreas

Digestive juices, including hydrochloric acid, pancreatin and pepsin, along with bile, decrease with age, these digestive juices may be inhibited by a lack of nutritional building blocks, medications, antibiotics that change the bacterial makeup of the digestive tract. Retinitis pigmentosa patients may wish to undergo evaluation for a digestive enzyme deficiency which may be interfering with the absorption of nutrients that are essential for retinal health. Since the cause of RP has eluded discovery within the eye, researchers might be wise to examine the metabolic pathways that may interfere with normal retinal nutrition.

A nutritional approach to gyrate atrophy

Gyrate atrophy is a rare retinal disorder. The successful treatment of gyrate atrophy by nutritional means provides hope that there are other nutritional remedies for the family of RP disorders. Gyrate atrophy affects the blood layer (choroid) and light receptor layer (retina) at the back of the eyes, usually beginning in childhood and leading to loss of vision somewhere between the fourth and seventh decade of life. Researchers discovered these patients are missing an important enzyme which then results in the over-supply of ornithine, an amino acid, in the retina. A high carbohydrate very low protein diet, combined with supplements of vitamin B6 to naturally stimulate enzyme production, has been shown to be an effective treatment.[36] This is just another example of an eye disorder that starts in the digestive tract.

Nutrition and Leber's hereditary retinal dystrophy

Of particular interest is Leber's optic atrophy which often arises between the ages of 18 and 25, usually in males. People who are diagnosed with Leber's optic nerve degeneration are believed to be hereditarily prone to develop the disease but alcohol and tobacco use apparently cause this serious eye disorder to become manifest.[37] A genetic defect in the mitochondria of the cells of the optic nerve is involved in Leber's disease.[38] (The mitochondria is the part of a living cell that produces energy.) Leber's disease does not always progress to severe loss of vision. Between 4 and 37 percent of Leber's patients experience visual recovery.[39] A blood test is now available to confirm the diagnosis of Leber's.[40] Coenzyme Q10 is the natural antioxidant for the cellular mitochondria[41] Supplements of coenzyme Q10 (30-100 mg.) could be helpful for people who have Leber's disease.

Researchers also believe Leber's disease is due to defective cyanide metabolism, a toxic substance that is produced in the blood stream of smokers. When Vitamin B12, which detoxifies cyanide, is administered to individuals with Leber's optic nerve disease, vision often improves. Adults with Leber's or any retinal disease might avoid foods that produce cyanide (almonds, milk, cabbage, some kinds of beans) and smoking. The dietary prescription to detoxify cyanide from the retina is to take 1000-1500 mcg. a day of Vitamin B12 and the sulfur containing amino acid N-acetyl cysteine, 800 mg. a day, and methionine, 600 mg. a day. Patients with Leber's retinal dystrophy did not show progression of their disease when taking these supplements.[42]

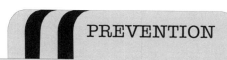

NUTRITION

PREVENTION

What are the preventive measures for RP?

Retinitis pigmentosa patients should do those things that make <u>common sense</u> and which in general are known to prevent visual loss and preserve or enhance night vision. These measures include good nutrition and protection from sun rays.

- Smoking tobacco is absolutely taboo for anyone who has a retinal disorder.

- Protect the eyes of RP patients from UV sun rays since these rays are known to promote cataracts, which are prevalent among anyone who is exposed daily to unfiltered sun rays.

- For comfort RP patients should wear hats. A hat with a three-inch brim provides adequate shade for the eyes and reduces the heat rays from direct overhead sun.

- Avoid alcohol, to keep the liver healthy, which is important for vitamin A production and metabolism.

- Eat a low fat diet, since a high fat diet has been linked with progression of RP. Saturated fats are also difficult for the pancreas to handle. The pancreas secretes bile that is needed for absorption of vitamin A.

- Supplement the diet with sources of omega-3 fatty acids. Walnuts, flax and cold-water fish (cod, salmon, tuna) are good sources of omega-3. Supplements containing both of these oils may be considered.

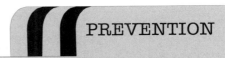

NUTRITION   PREVENTION

- RP patients, from early youth, should supplement their diet with vitamin A, beta carotene, all of the B vitamins (especially vitamin B12, thiamine, folic acid and vitamin B6), zinc, amino acids taurine and N-acetyl cysteine, vitamin E, vitamin C and bioflavonoids. These nutrients are known to be helpful in preventing cataracts which are common among RP patients.

- RP patients should undergo evaluation of their digestive system, to make sure their liver and pancreas are healthy. Digestive supplements of bile and other enzymes required to absorb and metabolize vitamin A may be recommended by a doctor.

- Foods that contain beta carotene should be plentiful in the diet. Sweet potatoes and carrots contain a form of beta carotene known as cis beta carotene that is easily absorbed. A small amount of fat and zinc is required in order to absorb and convert beta carotene into vitamin A. Thus beta carotene rich foods should be eaten with the meal that likely contains these other factors. Vegetarians will have less fat in their diet and may need to put a small amount of olive oil in with their foods to maximize beta carotene absorption.

- Avoid artificial fats (hydrogenated fats) found in margarines, baked goods, artificial eggs, and many other products.

- Zinc supplementation should not exceed 25 mg. per day since larger amounts rob the body of copper and may increase cholesterol levels.[43]

- Beta carotene capsules are absorbed better than eating carrots because the fiber (phytate) content of carrots

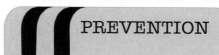

NUTRITION

PREVENTION

causes beta carotene to wash through the digestive tract.

- Vitamin A needs to be protected by other antioxidant vitamins or it will oxidize and be lost during absorption. Vitamin A is protected by vitamin E and vitamin E is protected by vitamin C. There is a synergistic effect when antioxidant vitamins are taken together.[44] The single vitamin approach to RP should be avoided since nutrients work together in the body and eyes.

- The goal of these measures is to slow down the progression of RP so that individuals can lead a near-normal life.

- To assist RP patients in finding brand names of vitamins that may be helpful the following nutritional formulas as recommended:

⇒ Take 4 capsules of Maxilife CoQ10 formula by Twinlab daily.

⇒ In addition to the above take 400 units of vitamin E daily and 1000 milligrams of taurine daily.

⇒ Take 1500 mcgs. of vitamin B12 daily. Many brands are available. Under-the-tongue caplets are available.

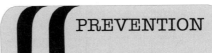

NUTRITION

PREVENTION

⇒ Take 500 milligrams of omega-3 fish oils from flax seed daily. There are many good brands available at your health food store.

⇒ Take 1-2 capsules of Super Enzyme Caps by Twinlab if indigestion or gas chronically occurs following meals. This formula includes all of the important digestive supplements. Only take this formula with meals, not on an empty stomach. The acid in these capsules can eat away the enamel on your teeth. Swallow the capsules, don't chew them. Digestive enzymes should not be taken by those who have stomach ulcers. Check with your physician before taking enzymes.

David A. Newsome M.D., has listed some "therapies" that have been used for retinitis pigmentosa:[45]

Anticoagulants
Bee stings, venom
Cyclodialysis
Diet
DMSO (dimethyl sulfoxide)
Electricity
ENKAD (yeast RNA hydrolysate)
Exercise

Hormonal preparations (thyroid, gonadal, pituitary)
Hyaluronidase

Light deprivation (tinted lenses)
Mineral supplements
Miotics
Placental implants, injections
Radiotherapy
Retinal and other tissue extracts (liver, pituitary)

Scleral trephination
Steroids
Sympathectomy, stellate ganglion blockage
Taurine
Transfer factor
Trephination
Ultrasound
Vasodilation
Vitamins, various
Zinc

REFERENCES

[1] Heckenlively J.R., RETINITIS PIGMENTOSA, J.B. Lippincott, Philadelphia 1988.

[2] Gouras P, et al, "Retinitis pigmentosa in abetalipoproteinemia: effects of vitamin A," Invest. Ophthalmology 10: 784-93, 1971.

[3] Boughman J., et al, "Population genetic studies of retinitis pigmentosa," Am. Journal Human Genetics 32: 223-35, 1980.

[4] Van Den Berg T.J.T.P., "Red glasses and visual function in retinitis pigmentosa," Documenta Ophthalmologica 73: 255-74, 1990.

[5] Newsome D.A., BlacharskiP., "Fundus flavimaculatus and retinitis pigmentosa," in RETINAL DISEASES, Mark O.M. Tso, Lippincott, Philadelphia 1988.

[6] Fusi, L., "Results show drug may slow progress of RP," Ophthalmology Times, August 1, 1991.

[7] Humphries P., "Gene located for retinitis pigmentosa," Genetic Technology News, August 1989.

[8] Bok D., "Retinal degeneration prevented in animal model," Ocular Surgery News, September 1, 1992, p. 31.

[9] Wofford D., "Saving sight," Winston-Salem Journal, September 29, 1988.

[10] Griggolo, F.M., "Night vision goggles for RP patients," Investigative Ophthalmology 34: ARVO Abstracts 1815-7, March 15, 1993.

[11] Heckenlively J.R., "Simplex retinitis pigmentosa," in RETINITIS PIGMENTOSA, J.B. Lippincott, Philadelphia, 1988, p. 192.

[12] Fishman G., "Thorough eye exams advised prior to taking two medications," Ophthalmology Times, January 1, 1983, pp. 1 & 64.

[13] Newsome D.A., et al, "Clinical and serum lipid findings in a large family with autosomal dominant retinitis pigmentosa," Ophthalmology 95: 1691-95, 1988.

[14] Weiter J., "Phototoxic changes in the retina," CLINICAL LIGHT DAMAGE TO THE EYE, Springer-Verlag, New York 1987.

[15] Leopold I.H., "Zinc deficiency and visual impairment?," American Journal of Ophthalmology 85: 871-75, 1978.

[16] Anderson R.E., et al, "Polyunsaturated fatty acids of photoreceptor membranes," Experimental Eye Research 18: 205-13, 1974.

[17] Converse C.C., et al, "Plasma lipid abnormalities in retinitis pigmentosa," Transactions Ophthalmic Society United Kingdom 103: 508-12, 1983.

[18] Herron W.L., Jr., "The dystrophic rat as a model for clinical research," in RETINITIS PIGMENTOSA, Plenum Press, New York, 1977, p. 145.

[19] Campbell D.A, Tonks E.L., "Biochemical findings in human retinitis pigmentosa with particular relation to vitamin A deficiency," British Journal Ophthalmology 46: 151-64, 1962.

[20] Campbell A.C., "Some physiological aspects of retinitis pigmentosa in man and animals," Transactions Ophthalmological Societies of U.K., 82: 667-702, 1963.

[21] Karcioglu Z.A., Stout R, Hahn H.J., "Serum zinc levels in retinitis pigmentosa," Current Eye Research 3: 1043-48, 1984.

[22] Karcioglu Z.A., "Low zinc levels noted in retinitis pigmentosa," Ophthalmology Times, January, 15, 1984, p. 5-6; Silverstone B.Z., et al, "Plasma zinc levels in high myopia and retinitis pigmentosa," Metabolic and Pediatric Ophthalmology 5: 187-90, 1981.

[23] Shearer A.C.I., "Absorption of B-carotene in human retinitis pigmentosa," Experimental Eye Research 3: 427-38; 1964.

[24] Berson E.L., et al, "A randomized trial of vitamin A and vitamin E supplementation for retinitis pigmentosa," Archives of Ophthalmology 111: 761-72, June 1993.

[25] Editorial, "Supplemental vitamin A retards loss of ERG amplitude in retinitis pigmentosa," Archives of Ophthalmology 111: 751-54, 1993.

[26] Rodger F.C., "Further study of the relation of vitamin A to retinal degenerations," Transactions Ophthalmological society U.K., 98: 128-133, 1978.

[27] Campbell A., MacEwen C.G., "Systemic treatment of Sjogrens Syndrome with Efamol (evening primrose oil), vitamin C and pyridoxine," in CLINICAL USES OF ESSENTIAL FATTY ACIDS, D.F. Horrobin, Eden Press, 1982.

[28] Itin P., Buchner S.A., Gloor B., "Darier's disease and retinitis pigmentosa; is there a pathological relationship?," British Journal of Dermatology 119: 397-402, 1988.

[29] Ennis S.R., Patulier E.L., "Retardation of inherited retinal dystrophy in the rat," Metabolic Pediatric Ophthalmology 3: 5-9, 1979.

pathological relationship?," British Journal of Dermatology 119: 397-402, 1988.

[29] Ennis S.R., Patulier E.L., "Retardation of inherited retinal dystrophy in the rat," Metabolic Pediatric Ophthalmology 3: 5-9, 1979.

[30] Pasantes-Morales H., et al, "Therapeutic effects of taurine and vitamin E in retinitis pigmentosa," in THERAPY WITH AMINO ACIDS AND ANALOGUES, First International Congress, Vienna, August 7-12, 1989.

[31] Rapp L.M., et al, "Synergism between environmental lighting and taurine depletion in causing photoreceptor cell degeneration," Experimental Eye Research 46: 229-38, 1988.

[32] Cogan D.G., et al, "Ocular abnormalities in abetalipoproteinemia; a clinicopathologic correlation," Ophthalmology 91: 991, 1984.

[33] Berger A.S., Tychsen L., Rosenblum J.L., "Retinopathy in human vitamin E deficiency," American Journal of Ophthalmology 111: 774-75, 1991.

[34] Pizzorno J., Murray M., ENCYCLOPEDIA OF NATURAL MEDICINE, Prima Publishing, Rocklin, Ca. 1990, p. 53.

[35] Newsome D.A., "Laboratory and diagnostic studies as adjuncts to the evaluation of retinal dystrophies and degenerations," RETINAL DSYTROPHIES AND DEGENERATIONS, David A. Newsome, editor, Raven Press, 1988, p. 71.

[36] Kaiser-Kupfer M.I., Caruso R.C., Valle D., "Gyrate atrophy of the choroid and retina," Archives of Ophthalmology, 109: 1539-48, 1991.

[37] Cullom, M.E., et al, "Leber's hereditary optic neuropathy masquerading as tobacco-alcohol amblyopia," Archives of Ophthalmology 111: 1482-85, 1993.

[38] Ortiz R.G., et al, "Variable retinal and neurologic manifestations in patients harboring the mitochondrial DNA 8993 mutation," Archives of Ophthalmology 111: 1525-30, 1993.

[39] Heher K.L., Johns D.R., "A maculopathy associated with the 15257 mitochondrial DNA mutation," Archives of Ophthalmology 111: 1495-99, 1993.

[40] Mackey D, Nasioulas S, Forrest S., "Finger prick blood testing in Leber hereditary optic neuropathy," British Journal of Ophthalmology 77: 311-12, 1993.

[41] Leibovitz B., "Coenzyme Q10," Nutrition Update 3: 1-9, Advanced Research Press, 1988.

[42] Cotticelli L, et al, "Red cell glutathione in Leber's Optic Atrophy," Metabolic Pediatric and Systemic Ophthalmology 8: 31-34, 1985.

[43] McClain C.J., Stuart M.A., "Zinc metabolism in the elderly," in GERIATRIC NUTRITION, John E. Morley, editor, Raven Press, New York, 1990.

[44] Wheater C., BETA CAROTENE, Thorsons, London, 1991.

[45] Newsome D.A., RETINAL DYSTROPHIES AND DEGENERATIONS, Raven Press, New York 1988.

Quick facts

<u>*Part of the eye affected*</u>*-- vitreous*

<u>*Typical age of onset*</u>*-- age 60 for normal eyes; any age for nearsighted or migrainous eyes*

<u>*Risk factors*</u>*-- diabetes, myopia, contact sports like boxing*

<u>*Modern treatment*</u>*-- removal of the vitreous can be performed, though this is not commonly performed*

<u>*Preventive measures*</u>*-- UV-blocking sunglasses, nutrition*

<u>*Questions to ask your eye doctor:*</u>
Does diet affect flashes and floaters?
Are floaters age-related?
How often should I schedule an eye exam?

4
FLOATERS AND FLASHES

What are floaters?

Floaters are clumps of protein that have formed within the jelly-like vitreous of the eye.   Floaters appear as shadows, cob webs, and flashing lights that occur when the vitreous jelly that fills the eyes detaches from the back (retina) of the eye.   While flashes of light and floaters usually do not signal a serious eye problem, sometimes they precede a retinal detachment and should always be checked by an ophthalmologist.

Are floaters a disease?

Most doctors consider the detachment of the jelly-like vitreous from the retina as a natural occurrence that cannot be prevented. Factors such as nutrition and sun exposure may affect the rate of liquefaction (gel becomes watery) of the vitreous.   UV sun rays promote clumping of vitreous proteins.

How many develop floaters?

Vitreous floaters often accompany the liquefaction of the normally jelly-like vitreous that fills 65 percent of the eye cavity. Pathologists examined hundreds of eyes and discovered that in one out of four adults the vitreous jelly of one or both eyes had become partially or completely detached. Most vitreous detachments don't occur till the middle of the sixth decade of life.   Diabetes is the most common predisposing condition for vitreous detachment.[1] Myopic (nearsighted) individuals experience a vitreous detachment 10 years earlier than adults who don't wear eyeglasses.[2]

While a vitreous detachment is rare for persons under age 30, its prevalence increases to 10 percent in persons between 30 and 59,

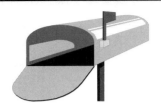

Mail bag

Please help! You are my last resort! My only remaining hope! 'It' occurred in my left eye initially... though it appears I don't have a hole or tear in my retina per se, the eye doctor was able to see my new , large and annoying floater, as well as the condition of my vitreous gel which appears to be 'ungelling' and causing flashes and floaters. What can be done to prevent further flashes and floaters from occurring? Is it possible to 're-gel' my vitreous?
K.O.
Pittsburgh, PA.

27 percent among persons between 60-69, and to 63 percent in persons over age 70.[3]   This explains why some relatively young adults complain of floaters.

What is it like to have floaters?

The typical individual who experiences floaters doesn't know what to think of these bothersome visual disturbances. One woman called her ophthalmologist's office and said *"Either my house is infested with gnats or I'm going blind."* The receptionist explained that the problem was probably vitreous floaters. When these clumps of protein get in the pathway of light as it enters the eyes they cast a shadow onto the retina. Most patients are frustrated and confused about floaters and wonder why there isn't something that can be done for them.

Flashes of light accompany floaters about a third of the time. People are more aware of these flashes in dim illumination.

Showers of floaters, "reddish smoke" or blurred vision signal a more serious vitreous hemorrhage that occurs among 13-19 percent of persons who experience an acute vitreous detachment.[4] As the vitreous peels away from the retina it may also cause a tear in the retina.

Once the vitreous has detached, an event which one will certainly be aware of because of floaters and flashes of light, you should be on the lookout for a "curtain" or "shadow" in your peripheral vision. This is often the first sign of a retinal detachment. This advice is especially important for individuals who are at a high risk to develop a retinal detachment such as diabetics and those who have moderate to severe amounts of myopia.

If floaters occur should a person schedule an eye exam?

The big question is, when are floaters nothing more than a harmless visual disturbance, and when do they signal that a retinal detachment or other eye problem is impending? In one study,

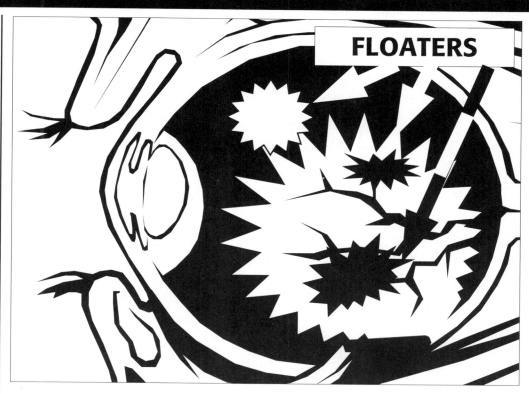

researchers found that 24 percent of patients who had multiple floaters had sight-threatening conditions, the most serious being retinal detachment. A single isolated floater was not considered serious enough to prompt an eye exam.[5]

Generally, no treatment is warranted for vitreous detachments. If they are accompanied by a tear in the retina or a retinal detachment, <u>then immediate treatment is needed.</u>

Can floaters be prevented?

Ultraviolet sun rays can promote the shrinkage and breakdown of the vitreous gel of the eye.[6] Frequently older adults experience more floaters following the removal of cataracts. This occurs because the vitreous gel of the eyes is exposed to more sun rays following cataract extraction.

Researchers discovered that a destructive variety of oxidation involving singlet oxygen is responsible for the breakdown of the vitreous.[7,8]

It is reasonable to believe that the wearing of totally UV-protective sunglasses could delay or prevent vitreous floaters. High intake of antioxidants, vitamin C, vitamin E, beta carotene, bioflavonoids, may slow down or prevent the progression of floaters. Because floaters occur more frequently among diabetics, control of blood sugar may also be helpful.

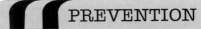

NUTRITION

PREVENTION

To prevent floaters:

Always wear 100 percent UV-filtering sunglasses when outdoors.

Take any of the following brands of antioxidant supplements:

⇒ Maxilife CoQ10 formula by Twinlab
⇒ Ocuguard by Twinlab
⇒ Vizion by Solaray
⇒ Protegra by Lederle
⇒ Ocucare by Nature's Plus

⇒ Take 1000-3000 milligrams of bilberry extract.

REFERENCES

[1] Foos R.Y., "Posterior vitreous detachment," Transactions American Academy of Ophthalmology and Otolaryngology 76: 480-97, 1972.
[2] Akiba J., "Prevalence of posterior vitreous detachment in high myopia," Ophthalmology, 100: 1384-88, 1993.
[3] Foos R.Y., Wheeler N.C., Vitreoretinal juncture: synchysis senilis and posterior vitreous detachment," Ophthalmology 89: 1502, 1982.
[4] Benson W.E., RETINAL DETACHMENT, 2nd edition, Lippincott, Philadelphia, 1980.
[5] Diamong J.P., "When are simple flashes and floaters ocular emergencies?," Eye 6: 102-04, 1992.
[6] Lerman S., RADIANT ENERGY AND THE EYE, Macmillan, New York, 1980, p. 164.
[7] Ueno N., Chakrabarti B., "UV light induced liquefaction and generation of damaging photosensitizer in the vitreous of simulated aphakic eyes," Investigative Ophthalmology 30: 62 ARVO Abstracts, March 15, 1989.
[8] Ueno N., et al, "Effects of visible-light irradiation on vitreous structure in the presence of a photosensitizer," Experimental Eye Research 44: 863-70, 1987.

Quick facts:

Part of the eye affected-- *retina*

Typical time of onset-- *any time after trauma (any blow to the eye or brow); any time following eye surgery; any time after age 30 in nearsighted patients*

Risk factors-- *myopia, contact sports (especially boxing)*

Modern treatment- *surgery*

Preventive measures-- *regular eye exams*

Questions to ask your eye doctor:

What are the signs and symptoms? How likely is it that the other retina will detach? Once repaired, can the retina detach again? How successful is retinal reattachment?

5
RETINAL DETACHMENT

"I lost an old friend the other day. He was blue eyed, impish, he cried a lot with me, laughed a lot with me, saw a great many things with me. I don't know why he left me.... We read a lot of books together.....we saw films together. He had a pretty exciting life. He saw Babe Ruth hit a home run when we were both 12 years old. He saw Willie Mays steal second base......... I thought he led a pretty good life.

You see, the friend I lost was my eye. I suppose I should be grateful that he didn't drift away when I was 12 or 15 or 29 but stuck around over 50 years until we had a vault of memories. Still, I'm only human. I'd like to see again."

-- Sports writer Jim Murray of the Los Angeles Times talking about his retinal detachment in July of 1979.

What is a retinal detachment?

A retinal detachment is when the layer of film that produces vision at the back of the eye detaches from the eye. About the size of a postage stamp, the retina can be torn or pulled from its normal position by changes within the jelly-like vitreous that fills the eyes.

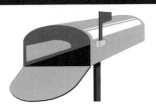

Mail Bag

My chropractor told me to take bilberry extract to help my eyes. I had a retinal detachment in my left eye which has been repaired. I have floaters sometimes in my other eye. Can retinal detachments reoccur? Is there anything that can be done to prevent them?

C.Q.
Omaha,
Nebraska

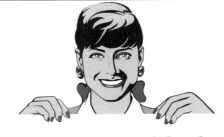

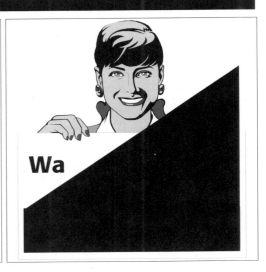

The most common retinal detachment appears as a black curtain in the lower field of view.

A retinal detachment requires immediate and urgent attention. Most people who experience this problem are slow to recognize that the "black curtain" in their vision is a retinal detachment.

How many experience retinal detachments?

People who are highly nearsighted or who have undergone cataract removal are more prone to develop retinal detachments. Boxers have a high rate of retinal detachment from repeated head trauma. Boxer Sugar Ray Leonard was forced into early retirement in 1982 when he suffered a retinal detachment. Each year over 200 retinal detachments are reported among boxers. Only 16 percent of retinal detachments are caused by head trauma.[1]

The incidence of retinal detachment of adults over age 50 is approximately 30 people per 100,000. According to the National Eye Institute, approximately 25,000 people suffer detached retinas annually in the U.S. Following treatment, 4,000 of these will have full vision restored, 15,000 will recover some vision, and 6,000 will lose a significant amount of their vision.

With immediate treatment there is a good prognosis that retinal detachment patients will not lose their sight, but 40 percent of the time vision isn't restored to 20/20.[2]

The degree of myopia increases the risk of retinal detachment. Mild amounts of nearsightedness (-1.00 to -.300 diopters) increase the risk by four times. More than -3.00 eyeglass prescriptions increase the risk of detachment by ten times.[3]

What is it like to experience a retinal detachment?

The typical patient doesn't seek attention fast enough and has floaters for weeks prior to their detachment. Wait too long and it can't be reattached; blindness is the result. A permanent veil that blocks part of your vision should not be ignored. A common occurrence is when the eye is hit by a blunt object, such as a racquetball, a fist, or any other object. The eye can be repaired within 48 hours of an event and the sooner the better. Every new onset of floaters should be seen by an ophthalmologist.

What is the modern treatment for retinal detachment?

The overall success rate of retinal re-attachment surgery is between 70 and 95 percent but a successful reattachment does not mean good vision is restored.

The retina can be gently reattached by indenting the wall of the eyes, like squeezing a tennis ball, and inducing the retina into place. Sewing a piece of silicone onto the wall of the eyes helps to push the retina closer to its normal position. This operation is called a scleral buckle.

Miniature balloons are sometimes placed next to the outer wall of the eye and inflated, thus thrusting the retina back into its normal position.[4]

Intense cold can be used to seal a retinal hole accompanying a retinal detachment. This technique is called cryopexy.

Another technique involves the instillation of silicone oil inside the vitreous cavity to press against the inner retina.

Eye surgeons can inject a gas that pushes the retina back in place.

Retinal surgeons may inject an inert gas into the eye to push the retina back in place. This technique is called pneumatic retinopexy and it has been shown to restore 20/50 vision or better to 71 percent of patients who have experienced a retinal detachment.[5]

Can retinal detachments be prevented?

Prompt attention to this condition when it occurs increases the chances of visual restoration. Patients who belong to health maintenance organizations often experience delays in treatment and this decreases the chance of sight restoration.

Highly myopic individuals are an "at risk" population to develop a retinal detachment. Anything that can be done to strengthen the thin retinal film at the back of the eyes may help to delay or prevent its occurrence.

Researchers have observed that the photosensitive chemicals in the retinal cells are decreased following retinal detachment. When retinal detachments were intentionally induced in animal eyes, the eyes that were kept in darkness were more normal than eyes that were exposed to light. Keeping the eyes in total darkness, or wearing dark sunglasses, may be helpful during the rehabilitation period following a retinal re-attachment operation.[6]

Low Vitamin A (beta carotene) levels have been suggested as a factor in retinal detachment and supplements may be advisable following a retinal detachment.[7]

Because retinal detachments are often preceded by flashes of light and showers of floaters, be aware of these symptoms. A mild floater that reoccurs from time to time should not be of concern. Neither should scintillating flashes of light that accompany migraines. As long as floaters last less than twenty minutes they usually do not represent vitreous detachment.

Once a retinal detachment has occurred, if vision is to be restored prompt examination and treatment by a retinal specialist is critical. Don't let anyone delay treatment for this problem.

REFERENCES

[1] King P., "How experts view Leonard's retina," Los Angeles Herald Examiner, May 11, 1982.
[2] Burton T.C., "Recovery of visual aucity after retinal detachment involving the macula," Transactions American Ophthalmological Society 70-475-97, 1982.
[3] Eye Disease Case Control Study Group, "Risk factors for idiopathic rhegmatogenous retinal detachment," American Journal of Epidemiology 137: 749-57, 1993.
[4] "Balloon reattaches retinas," Science Digest, May 1983, p. 89.
[5] Gribomont A., "Pneumatic retinopexy equally as effective as scleral buckling," Ophthalmology Times, September 15, 1991, p. 22.
[6] Charles S., Machemer R., "Experimental retinal detachment in the owl monkey," American Journal of Ophthalmology 78: 233-35, 1974.
[7] Dowlin J.E., Gibbons I.R., "The effect of vitamin A deficiency on the five structures of the retina; in THE STRUCTURE OF THE EYE, Smelser, Academic Press, New York, 1961.

Quick facts

Part of the eye affected-- retina and optic nerve

Typical age of onset-- older years

Risk factors-- high fat and cholesterol diet; vasospasm (constriction of muscles that control the diameter of blood vessels)

Modern treatment-- blood thinners, anti-cholesterol agents, calcium-channel blockers

Preventive measures: low-fat diets, exercise, smoking cessation, antioxidant supplements, omega-3 fatty acids, other supplements.

Questions to ask your eye doctor--

How low should my cholesterol level be?
How do I improve blood flow?

6

CIRCULATORY PROBLEMS OF THE RETINA AND OPTIC NERVE, OR HARDENING OF THE ARTERIES

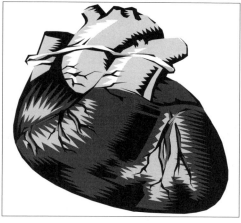

The eye is the only organ where the blood vessels can be examined directly under magnification. When the tiny blood vessels at the back of the eyes become diseased, clogged with fats, blocked by blood clots, obstructed by a buildup of calcifications and constricted by smooth muscle spasm, a host of eye problems can result. When blood vessel disease is observed during an eye examination it should warrant immediate changes in diet, exercise and nutrition. When physicians diagnose blood vessel disease in other parts of the body they define it as angina, thrombophlebitis, stroke, carotid artery disease, coronary artery disease and Raynaud's phenomenon. All doctors are doing is defining the location of the disease. Eye problems such as glaucoma and macular degeneration may occur sooner than other blood vessel problems because the small blood vessels at the back of the eyes may become occluded earlier than large vessels.

What is hardening of the arteries of the eyes?

Blood vessel disease in the eyes can be categorized as follows:

1. **Acute total blockage of blood vessels which may occur suddenly, resulting in retinal vein or artery occlusion and a sudden decrease in vision.** This may result from a blood clot, a fatty plug or calcific rock usually released from the heart or carotid

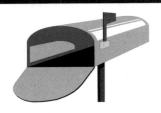

Mail bag

artery in the neck into the blood circulation. This condition often resolves within a few months as the blockage dissolves.[1]

2. **A sudden temporary blockage of a retinal blood vessel caused by vasospasm (blood vessel constriction) which results in a visual blackout for a few minutes** (called amaurosis fugax).[2]

3. **The gradual lifetime narrowing of the ocular blood vessels due to a combined buildup of fatty plaques (cholesterol), micro-blood clots, calcifications or vasospasm which results in glaucoma, macular degeneration or diabetic retinopathy.**[3]

What are the underlying causes of blood vessel disease?

Glaucoma, macular degeneration, diabetic retinopathy and retinal vein and artery occlusions all are accompanied by any combination of the following factors:

Reduced blood flow through the vessels[4,5]
Increased blood viscosity[6,7]
Increased total cholesterol, triglycerides and LDL cholesterol[8]
Increased lipoprotein (a)[9]
Clots elsewhere in the vascular system (heart, legs, brain)
Vasospasm (smooth muscle that lines the blood vessels constricts reducing the diameter of the vessels)[10]
Silent heart attacks[11]
High blood pressure
High fat diet[63]
Overweight[12]
Typical Western diet low in omega-3 fats[13]
High hematocrit (>50)[14]
High intracellular levels of calcium (promotes vasospasm)
Low magnesium[15]
Evidence of other vascular diseases (migraine, Raynaud's)[16]
Sedentary lifestyle

How many have diseased blood vessels in their eyes?

The answer to the above question is many millions of older Americans have diseased ocular blood vessels. In fact the hardening of the arteries is probably the primary underlying cause of three major eye disorders-- glaucoma, macular degeneration and diabetic retinopathy.

A report by the National Heart, Lung and Blood Institute compares

SIGHT LIMITATION WITH AND WITHOUT CARDIOVASCULAR DISEASE		
AGE GROUP	NO VASCULAR DISEASE	WITH VASCULAR DISEASE
65-74	5.1%	9.3%
75-84	11.5%	18.0%
85+	19.6%	38.5%

the incidence of sight limitation among senior adults who have blood vessel (vascular) disease with those who are free of disease. **This shocking report indicates blood vessel disease increases sight limitations by 56 to 96 percent among various groups of senior adults age 65 to 85+.**[17]

Patients who have diabetes, high blood pressure, high cholesterol levels, migraine and a host of other medical conditions, and who take oral contraceptives, have been shown to be prone to develop blockage of a central retinal blood vessel. Nearly half of these patients have carotid artery disease.

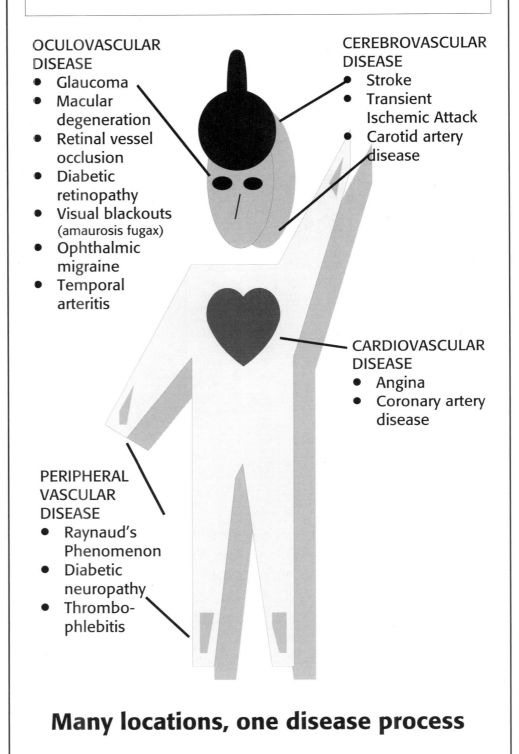

The Family of Blood Vessel Diseases

OCULOVASCULAR DISEASE
- Glaucoma
- Macular degeneration
- Retinal vessel occlusion
- Diabetic retinopathy
- Visual blackouts (amaurosis fugax)
- Ophthalmic migraine
- Temporal arteritis

CEREBROVASCULAR DISEASE
- Stroke
- Transient Ischemic Attack
- Carotid artery disease

CARDIOVASCULAR DISEASE
- Angina
- Coronary artery disease

PERIPHERAL VASCULAR DISEASE
- Raynaud's Phenomenon
- Diabetic neuropathy
- Thrombo-phlebitis

Many locations, one disease process

NUTRITIONAL ANTIDOTES FOR BLOOD VESSEL DISEASE

CHOLESTEROL 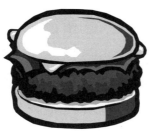	**Very low-fat diet** (10% saturated fat) **Antioxidants prevent cholesterol from hardening within blood vessels** ♦ **Vitamin E** ♦ **Vitamin C** ♦ **Beta carotene** ♦ **Bioflavonoids** ♦ **Garlic**
BLOOD CLOTS 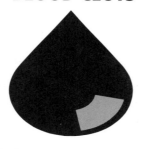	♦ **Omega-3 oils** ♦ **Garlic** ♦ **Magnesium** ♦ **Vitamn E**
CALCIFICATIONS 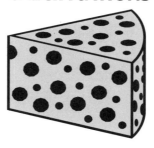	**Avoidance of excess calcium**
VASOSPASM 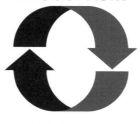	**Magnesium** (calcium channel blocker)

What is it like to have a blocked blood vessel at the back of the eyes?

Blockage of main blood vessels most commonly occurs between the ages of 50 and 70. The typical patient may notice a mild or severe blurring of vision, mainly in the center of their vision, that sometimes improves during the day. Night blindness and light sensitivity are other common symptoms. There may be multiple black spots, floaters and other abnormal visual sensations. Some patients may falsely believe they are hallucinating and are afraid or embarrassed to mention seeing flashes or floaters.[18] When the retina is deprived of oxygen, called ischemia, eye pain may occur in up to 40 percent of patients. This is experienced as a dull ache in and around the eyes.[19] Sometimes a migraine attack can be confused for a retinal vein or artery occlusion.

Are blood thinners helpful?

In the 1950's two studies were conducted using blood thinners to treat macular degeneration.

In the first study heparin, a blood thinner, was given intravenously to patients with macular degeneration in an attempt to clear their diseased retinal blood vessels and improve sight. The first report in 1957 showed the following results:[20]

⇒ 16 of the 24 macular disease patients showed mild to marked visual improvement following heparin treatment.

⇒ 3 cases were stable and only 3 cases were worse following heparin treatment.

This positive preliminary report was followed in 1959 by a study of 48 macular disease patients who underwent the same heparin therapy. The results of this second study were not as positive. Half of the 48 patients only received injections of salt water and yet nearly the same percentage claimed their vision improved as the patients who received the blood thinner. Here are the results of that study:[21]

Vision:	Same	Better	Worse
Heparin (blood thinner)	14	7	8
Salt water injection	10	8	6

Some of these elderly patients in this second study adamantly claimed that their vision improved following the salt water injections even though this was not demonstrated when their vision was tested. The researchers involved in this report concluded that the patients were *"unjustifiably optimistic about the improvement of their eyes."*

Another small group of macular disease patients given special medical attention, was grouped with other patients in a "support group" and was provided optimistic encouragement. They were compared with a small group of patients who were not given individual attention nor any encouragement and who tended to claim all sorts of undesirable symptoms from their treatment.

Despite the fact that extra attention and encouragement appeared to improve the subjective visual quality of these patients the doctors said *"we do not endorse giving ineffectual medications to the patients with senile macular degeneration."* The doctors suggested that a balanced diet, weight loss and exercise be recommended not because these suggestions helped the eyes but because they *"give the patient something to do for himself."*

Largely because of this second report the use of blood thinners was abandoned.

The conclusions of these reports need to be scrutinized.

1. The doctors failed to give any credence to the role of positive mental attitude, stress reduction and possible resultant reduction in blood vessel spasm.

2. The fact that some patients' vision improved, as documented by these doctors themselves, proves that macular degeneration does not always become progressively worse. There are factors that cause this disease to wax and wane.

3. There was too much reliance upon visual acuity or visual field tests which are only two measures of visual quality. Color vision and contrast vision (ability to see shades of grey) were not measured even though they are known to be affected by macular disease. The subjective improvements noted by these patients may have gone unmeasured.

4. Patients who are given some control over an otherwise untreatable disease have been given hope for their condition. While doctors should not promise false cures for their patients neither should they suggest that their patients give up all hope of seeing again.

5. Some of the patients who received heparin therapy experienced bleeding problems. The use of milder blood thinners (such as garlic and omega-3 fatty acids) may be safer and more effective.

6. These studies conducted in the 1950's failed to consider the combined effect of the four main causes of ocular blood vessel disease--- fatty plaques, blood clots, calcifications and vasospasm. These doctors errantly believed that heparin reduces fatty plaques within blood vessels when heparin is known to reduce the aggregation of blood platelets that promote blood clots.

What treatments are available?

Because eye physicians are often unable to determine the exact cause of the blockage of the retinal blood vessels, there is little help available as far as treatment. Sometimes surgery is performed on the carotid artery, the principal artery in the neck. Steroids that help to reduce inflammation have been tried with little success. Anticoagulant therapy, blood thinning drugs such as heparin, have been suggested and have resulted in moderate to major improvement. Clot busting drugs, such as streptokinase and tissue plasminogen activator, have been tried to no avail. Aspirin and persantine are anti-platelet medications that keep the blood from sticking but have also been met with failure. About three to six months following a retinal vein occlusion, vision may spontaneously improve.[22]

Because blockage of the retinal blood arteries deprives the retinal cells of oxygen, new unwanted blood vessels may develop, a condition called neovascularization.   Placing vein occlusion patients in a hyperbaric oxygen chamber has been shown to temporarily improve vision among those who have mild ischemia (oxygen deprivation).[23]

What causes blood vessel disease?

There are five major reasons why small blood vessels in the retina become occluded:

Blood clots

1. Small clots or thrombi may develop as the blood thickens and platelets (clotting factors) in the blood clump together. The blood can become very thick.[24] This can be likened to oil for your car. Thin oil is 15 weight, while heavy oil has a viscosity of 40 or 50. The retinal blood vessels are among the smallest in the body, and if clots develop like sludge in your car's engine, vision can be affected. Retinal vein occlusions are usually caused by blood clots.[25]

The thickness (viscosity) of blood can range from 7 to 100 times thicker than water within the retina. A blood test, called a hematocrit which measures the volume of red blood cells in whole blood, can tell your eye doctor if your blood is too thick. A hematocrit exceeding 50 indicates your blood is too thick.[26]

Cholesterol

2. A buildup of cholesterol (fats) and triglycerides has been shown to narrow the retinal blood vessels over time. Many of the patients with this condition have underlying high blood pressure, diabetes and may require measures to control blood sugar and hypertension.[27]

Blood vessel spasm

3. Blood vessels may spasm, a condition called vasospasm.   The blood vessels are not just a limp hose, they are lined with muscle that can constrict or dilate their inner diameter.

Calcifications

4. Calcification of the blood vessel walls.[28]

Carotid artery obstruction

5. Poor blood flow to the retina may occur when the carotid artery, the primary artery in the neck, becomes occluded. It is believed that the narrowing of the carotid artery may deprive the retina of oxygen and result in the development of new unwanted blood vessels inside the eye. This can cause neovascular glaucoma, neovascular diabetic retinopathy, and neovascular "wet" macular degeneration. Patients who describe episodes of visual loss in one eye, lasting for a few seconds to several minutes, often have a narrow carotid artery.[29]

Patients with narrowed carotid arteries should employ many of the healthful measures outlined in this book rather than just believing that an operation to clean out the carotid artery will fix their problem. The number of carotid artery surgeries, called endarterectomy, has increased in recent years without clear evidence that the operation is helpful.[30]

A combination of two or more of the above factors are likely involved in most cases of occlusive retinal blood vessel disease. When cholesterol plaques combine with blood clots a temporary occlusion of the artery is more likely.

It is likely that all of the above factors play a role in occlusive vascular retinal disease. The necessity to treat all these factors is a probable reason why attempts to treat this emergent eye problem with one type of therapy haven't proven to be effective.

Lipoprotein (a)

While American doctors and their patients have become familiar with terms such as cholesterol and triglycerides, they may not be acquainted with another measure of fats in the blood stream called lipoprotein (a). This is a protein substance bound to a fat molecule. Patients with abnormally high lipoprotein (a) in their blood stream have been shown to be at risk to develop retinal vein occlusion as well as coronary heart disease and stroke. Only three compounds have been identified that reduce lipoprotein (a). Two of these, an anabolic steroid and high doses of niacin, have side effects. Omega-3 fatty acids, found in fish oils such as cod liver oil or flax seed oil, have been used for many decades and if taken in the proper dosages are relatively free of side effects.[31] Hopefully, the supplementation of omega-3 fats in the diet can help patients with occlusive retinal blood vessel disorders recover their sight.

Aspirin and retinal diseases

When mega-doses (500 milligrams a day) of aspirin are taken the ophthalmic artery blood flow improves by widening of the carotid artery.[32] However, aspirin has other adverse side effects and is not recommended for any individual with retinal diseases. Omega-3 fatty acids, garlic, magnesium and vitamin E may be safer and more effective.

Are blood vessel diseases well understood?

It has been said that doctors over-diagnose health problems but often have little to offer in the way of treatment. The following quote was made concerning strokes:

> *"What is painfully obvious to experts on stroke is that we still don't know which patients, with what lesions, detected by which tests, should be treated with what therapies."*[33]

Just like strokes, eye physicians are oftentimes puzzled as to how to treat blood vessels, located deep inside the eyes, that have a circumference no bigger than twine.

The eye's cholesterol meter

Which of the following is the best indicator of an increased risk of experiencing a future heart attack?

  1. High blood pressure
  2. High cholesterol
  3. Cigarette smoking

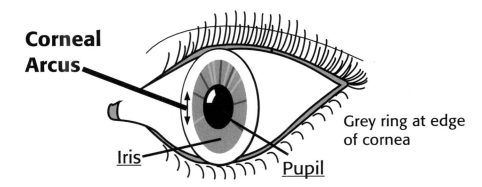

Corneal Arcus

Iris

Pupil

Grey ring at edge of cornea

4. A grey ring encircling the cornea of the eyes

For men under age 50 the presence of arcus may be a better indicator that they are at risk of having a heart attack than a blood cholesterol test or any of the other risk factors listed above.[34] Men with this sign have a 2 to 4 times increased likelihood they would die of a heart attack than men without this indication.

The presence of a grey ring at the outer edge of the clear cornea is a condition known as arcus. The cornea is the clear front window of the eyes. The intake of fats is so high in this country that the presence of arcus in the general population ranges from 25 to 35 percent and increases with age.[35] It occurs more frequently in men, who are known to have a higher rate of heart disease than women. One study found that 100 percent of adults have arcus by age 80.[36]

The grey ring is composed of fats accumulating in the body. The appearance of a grey ring in the cornea has been reproduced in animals by feeding them large doses of cholesterol. At the same time, the animals developed plaques in the arteries throughout their bodies.

Magnesium overcomes vasospasm

When vasospasm of the retinal blood vessels occurs supplementation of magnesium in the diet may be helpful. Daily magnesium supplements have been shown to relieve spasms of retinal blood vessels.[40] Magnesium relaxes smooth muscles found in the heart and blood vessels and opposes the action of calcium which promotes constriction of blood vessels. Magnesium, an essential mineral that is lacking in the western diet, is known as

The body has a way of visibly indicating abnormally high intake of saturated fats in our diets. Adults with corneal arcus have a nine in ten chance that their cholesterol exceeds 200 mg/dL.[37] A study published in the Journal of the American Medical Association shows that American men ages 35-57 years are at an increased risk for coronary heart disease if their cholesterol exceeds 180 mg/dL.[38]

It has been discovered that nearly two-thirds of the adults who exhibit arcus have marked arteriosclerosis in their retinal blood vessels at the back of their eyes while only one-third of adults without arcus show the same problem.[39] The eye is the window to the body.

nature's calcium channel blocker. Low magnesium levels have been found in 30 percent of diabetics who are prone to develop blockage of their retinal blood vessels.[41] Restoring magnesium levels in the body has been shown to decrease the risk of sudden cardiac arrest and coronary heart disease.[42]

Vasospasm is believed to be a primary cause of low-pressure glaucoma and migraines. Many of these patients have cold hands due to poor circulation. When the hands of low-pressure glaucoma patients are dipped in cold water the visual field is narrowed.[43]

Eye physicians will be tempted to perform blood tests for magnesium levels among patients with retinal vein or artery occlusion. Only tissue levels of magnesium, not serum levels, provide accurate information as to whether patients are deficient in this important mineral.

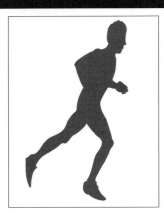

Physical exercise is important. Even a daily routine of brisk walking can yield big dividends in health maintenance.

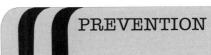

NUTRITION

PREVENTION

What is the recommended nutritional regimen for hardening of the blood vessels of the eyes?

☐ Eat a very low-fat diet by eliminating or minimizing saturated fats from meat and dairy product in the diet. Replace with fresh fruits and vegetables.

☐ For a fresh vein occlusion take 2500 mg. of omega-3 oil from flax seed daily. When the visual problem improves reduce the dosage of daily omega-3 oils to 500 mg. Only take under the direction of a physician. Do not take more omega-3 oils than recommended.

☐ Concern has been expressed about an increased risk of bleeding after intake of omega-3 fats, but the risk seems to be very low and is considered less than that posed by the intake of aspirin.[44] Up to 2500 mg. of omega-3 can be taken without adversely affecting blood sugar or cholesterol profiles.[45]

☐ For macular degeneration and glaucoma, refer to the nutritional suggestions in other sections of this book.

☐ Macular degeneration may require months of nutritional supplementation before any improvement is noticed in vision. Only take these supplements under the watchful direction of your eye physician. Do not take anything that thins the blood if already on Warfarin or Coumadin. Follow the nutritional suggestions in the section of this book under macular degeneration.

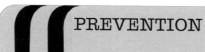

☐ Cease smoking and avoid caffeine which promotes vasospasm.

☐ Start a walking, aerobic exercise, bicycling or swimming program.

☐ Avoid calcium supplements that do not also include magnesium. Calcium promotes constriction of blood vessels. Take supplements that provide a 50-50 ratio of calcium and magnesium.

☐ Use every means available to reduce stress in your life through prayer and relaxation techniques. Stress increases vasospasm.

☐ **No promises can be made that vision will return to normal by following the above regimen and some people may experience minor side effects.** Always consult with a physician and seek out other sources of information before starting a new health regimen.

Apparently Western medical doctors have much to learn about this type of eye disorder. In China, eye physicians used a combination of herbs to improve blood circulation and thin the blood. They were able to stabilize or slightly improve vision among 84 percent of patients who had experienced a retinal vein occlusion. Nearly all of these patients had already been treated with Western drugs, which had little benefit.[46] It should be noted that 60 percent of patients with retinal vein occlusion recover at least to 20/40 vision or better within a year of their blockage, even without treatment.[47]

Eye physicians will be tempted to perform blood tests for magnesium levels among patients with retinal vein or artery occlusion. Only tissue levels of magnesium, not serum levels, provide accurate information as to whether patients are deficient in this important mineral.

REFERENCES

[1] Hollenhorst, R.W., "Significance of bright plaques in the retinal arterioles," Journal American Medical Association 178: 23-29, October 7, 1961.
[2] Winterkorn, J.M.S., et al, "Brief report: treatment of vasospastic amaurosis fugax with calcium-channel blockers," New England Journal of Medicine 329:396, 1993.
[3] Gasser, P., "Ocular vasospasm: a risk factor in the pathogenesis of low-tension glaucoma," International Ophthalmology 13: 281-90, 1989.
[4] Langham M.E., et al, "Blood flow in the human eye," Acta Ophthalmologica Supplementum 191, 67: 9-13, 1989.
[5] Rimmer T., et al, "Long-term follow-up of retinal blood flow in diabetes using the blue light entoptic phenomenon," British Journal of Ophthalmology 73: 1-5, 1989.
[6] Klaver, J.H.J., Greve E.L., Goslinga H., Geissen, H.C., Heuvelmans J.H.A., "Blood and plasma viscosity measurements in patients with glaucoma," British Journal of Ophthalmology 69: 765-70, 1985.
[7] Greve E.L. "Glaucoma: mechanical or vascular pathogenesis?," International Ophthalmology 16: 63, 1993.
[8] Winder A.F., "Circulating lipoprotein and blood glucose levels in association with low-tension and chronic simple glaucoma," British Journal of Ophthalmology 61: 641-45, 1977.
[9] Muller H.M., et al, "Lipoprotein (a): a risk factor for retinal vascular occlusion," German Journal of Ophthalmology 1: 338-41, 1992.
[10] Gasser P., Flammer J., "Influence of vasospasm on visual function," Documenta Ophthalmologica 66: 3-18, 1987.
[11] Kaiser, H.J., Flammer J., Burckardt, D., "Silent myocardial ischemia in glaucoma patients," Ophthalmologica 207: 6-8, 1993.
[12] Shiose, Y., "Intraocular pressure: new perspectives," Survey of Ophthalmology 34: 413-35, 1990.
[13] Schmidt E.B., Dyerberg J., "Omega-3 fatty acids," Drugs 47: 405-24, 1994.
[14] Foulds, W.S., "Blood is thicker than water: some haemorheological aspects of ocular disease," Eye 1: 343-63, 1987.
[15] White J.R., Jr., Campbell, R.K., "Magnesium and diabetes: a review," The Annals of Pharmacotherapy 27: 775-80, 1993.
[16] Phelps C.D., Corbett, J.J., "Migraine and low-tension glaucoma," Investigative Ophthalmology and Visual Science 26: 1105-08, 1985.
[17] Bild, D.E., et al, "Age-related trends in cardiovascular morbidity and physical functioning in the elderly: the cardiovascular health study," Journal American Geriatrics Society 41: 1047-56, 1993.
[18] Delaney W.V., "Ocular vascular disease: In-office primary care diagnosis," Geriatrics 48: 60-69, 1993.
[19] Madonna R.J., "Optometry and the carotid artery," Journal of the American Optometric Association, 64: 390-402, 1993.
[20] Rome, S., "Heparin in senile macular degeneration," A.M.A. Archives of Ophthalmology 57: 190-99, 1957.
[21] Havener W.H., Sheets J., Cook M.J., "Evaluation of heparin therapy of senile macular degeneration," A.M.A. Archives of Ophthalmology 61: 390-401, 1959.
[22] Fong A.C.O., Schatz H., "Central retinal vein occlusion in young adults," Survey of Ophthalmology 37: 393-417, 1993.
[23] Miyamoto H., Ogura Y., Honda Y., "Long term results of hyperbaric oxygen therapy for macular edema after retinal vein occlusion," Investigative Ophthalmology ARVO Abstracts 34: 685-25, March 15, 1993.
[24] Hayasaka S., et al, "Central retinal vein occlusion in two patients with immunoglobin G multiple myeloma associated with blood hyperviscosity," Annals of Ophthalmology 25: 191-94, 1993.

[25] Tso M.O.M., RETINA DISEASES, J.B. Lippincott, Philadelphia, 1988, p. 151.

[26] Foulds W.S., "Blood is thicker than water, Some haemorheological aspects of ocular disease," Eye 1: 343-63, 1987.

[27] Dodson P.M., Galton D.J., Hamilton A.M., Blach R.K., "Retinal vein occlusion and the prevalence of lipoprotein abnormalities," British Journal of Ophthalmology 66: 161-64, 1982.

[28] Younge B.R., "The significance of retinal emboli," Journal of Clinical Neuro-Ophthalmology 9: 190-4, 1989.

[29] Dugan J.D., Green W.R., "Ophthalmologic manifestations of carotid occlusive disease," Eye 5: 226-38, 1991.

[30] Cebul R.D., Whisnant J.P., "Carotid endarterectomy," Annals Internal Medicine 111: 660-70, 1989.

[31] Muller H.M., et al, "Lipoprotein (a): a risk factor for retinal vascular occlusion," German Journal of Ophthalmology 1: 338-41, 1992.

[32] Kana J.S., Horst G., Keller-Jentsen S., "Effect of long-term aspirin therapy on ophthalmic artery blood flow in patients with carotid atherosclerotic disease," Investigative Ophthalmology, ARVO Abstracts, 34: 3410-20, March 15, 1993.

[33] Caplan L.R., "Carotid artery disease," New England Journal of Medicine 315: 686-8, 1986.

[34] Edwards L.R., "Corneal arcus may be predictor of heart attack in some patients," Ophthalmology Times, June 15, 1988, p. 32.

[35] Barchiesi B.J., Eckel R.H., Ellis P.P., "The cornea and disorders of lipid metabolism," Survey of Ophthalmology 36: 1-22, 1991.

[36] Friedlander M.H., Smolin G., "Corneal degenerations," Annals Ophthalmology 11: 1486-95, 1979.

[37] Nishimoto J.H., et al, "Corneal arcus as an indicator of hypercholesterolemia," Journal American Optometric Association 61: 44-49, 1990.

[38] Stamler J., Wentworth D., Neaton J.D., "Is relationship between serum cholesterol and risk of premature death from coronary disease continuous and graded?," Journal American Medical Association 256: 2823-8, 1986.

[39] Caradonna B., "The corneal arcus reviewed," Townsend Letter for Doctors, July 1992, pp. 668-72.

[40] Cohen L, Laor A, Kitzes R., "Reversible retinal vasospasm in magnesium-treated hypertension despite no significant change in blood pressure," Magnesium 3: 159-63, 1984.

[41] Rude R.K., "Magnesium deficiency and diabetes mellitus," Postgraduate Medicine 92: 217-24, 1992.

[42] Singh R.B., "Effect of dietary magnesium supplementation in the prevention of coronary heart disease and sudden cardiac death," Magnesium Trace Elements 9: 143-51, 1990.

[43] Gasser P., Flammer J., "Influence of vasospasm on visual function," Documenta Ophthalmologica 66: 3-18, 1987.

[44] Leaf, A., Weber P.C., "Cardiovascular effects of n-3 fatty acids," New England Journal of Medicine 318: 549-57, 1988.

[45] Axelrod L., "Effects of a small quantity of w-3 fatty acids on cardiovascular risk factors in NIDDM," Diabetes Care 17: 37-44, 1994.

[46] Xiaoshu L., Chunyuan L., "TCM treatment of retinal vein occlusion in 216 cases," Journal of Traditional Chinese Medicine 10: 106-110, 1990.

[47] Tso M.O.M., RETINAL DISEASES, J.B. Lippincott, Philadelphia, 1988, p. 153.

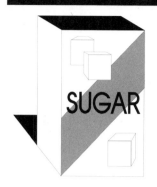

Despite the widespread use of sugar substitutes the consumption of refined sugar has increased in the U.S.

7
ARTIFICIAL SWEETENERS AND THE EYES

Lannie is a 40-year old woman who is diabetic. She carries around a bottle filled with a diet drink because she is continually thirsty. She has a severe case of glaucoma which has required various medications, laser treatment and surgery. She suffers with a chronic dry eye problem. Additionally, Lannie has been treated for chronic depression with Prozac, an antidepressant medication. Migraine headaches are another problem that Lannie has had to overcome.

Little did Lannie know that many of her health problems were related to side effects produced by continued daily ingestion of an artificial sweetener. Because of her diabetes Lannie had been advised to use non-sugar sweeteners. Aspartame (Nutrasweet) was taken daily when Lannie ate artificially sweetened yogurt, soft drinks, and other foods.

Of 6,000 complaints received by the Food and Drug Administration about adverse reactions to food ingredients, 80 percent were related to aspartame artificial sweetener and 15 percent to sulfite reactions.

There appears to be a segment of the population that experiences adverse reactions from ingestion of a high amount of aspartame sweetened foods and drinks. Like Lannie, most aspartame users are unaware of the potential side effects from overuse of artificial sweeteners.

It is reported that 5.8 pounds of aspartame sweetener is consumed annually per person in the U.S. As artificially sweetened drinks were promoted as a way of sparing calories and remaining slim, consumers began drinking more of these "non-fattening" beverages.

Some people have reported drinking up to 18 cans of aspartame sweetened cola drinks per day. Others continually "over-aspartame" themselves as aspartame is found in pre-sweetened tea, hot chocolate, chewing gum and coffee sweetener. Aspartame is now found in over 4,000 food products. It is a hidden ingredient in many non-sugar puddings, ice creams, and other desserts.

Aspartame actually appears to create a pseudo-dryness syndrome that makes a person thirsty, craving more and more fluids. Aspartame in some individuals appears to create a pseudo Sjogrens' Syndrome and should be avoided by those individuals who have arthritis or Sjogrens' Syndrome. [See the section in this series under dry eyes and Sjogrens' Syndrome.]

H.J. Roberts M.D. has compiled a complete book on the adverse health reactions related to aspartame. For those readers who are interested in reading more about this topic, pick up a copy of ASPARTAME (NUTRASWEET*): IS IT SAFE? Charles Press, Philadelphia 1990.

*A registered trademark of the Nutrasweet Company

Here are the most common health complaints ascribed to aspartame products:

- Severe headache. A dull headache can be experienced by many people shortly after ingesting an aspartame laced product.

- Seizures (convulsions)

- Impairment of vision. Twenty-five percent of aspartame users who report health problems report visual disturbances. Nine percent report unexplained eye pain, 8 percent report problems with contact lenses and 3 percent report loss of vision.

- Dizziness

- Atypical unexplained pain in various parts of the body -- the eyes, ears, face, neck

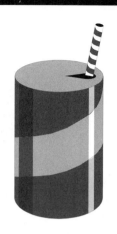

Aspartame is now found in over 4,000 food products

- Rashes

- Extreme fatigue

- Depression

- A change of personality

- Confusion and memory loss

The above information should not be construed to mean that moderate amounts of Nutrasweet aren't safe to use among healthy individuals. Nutrasweet has been approved by the FDA and has been judged to be relatively safe. From the information that Dr. H.J. Roberts and others have compiled, however, Nutrasweet is not totally safe for everyone.

What is it that makes aspartame a potential problem for the eyes?

Aspartame is made of up two amino acids or protein building blocks -- phenylalanine, aspartic acid, and methanol or wood alcohol. Methanol is the greatest cause for concern because it is a highly toxic agent to the optic nerve of the human eye. While the methanol content of aspartame is not large, it is the first component of the sweetener to be released within the upper small intestine and is readily absorbed.

The argument is that there is no more methanol in aspartame than found naturally in fruits and vegetables. The average daily intake of alcohol from natural sources is estimated at less than 10 milligrams, and is not as readily absorbed into the brain, eyes and other tissues as methanol found in aspartame.

Methanol (wood alcohol) is known to be toxic to the retina. Recently, an outbreak optic nerve blindness was reported in Cuba. This was eventually linked to home brewing of rum which contained methanol (wood alcohol) and very poor nutrition.[1] Many of the cases were due to vitamin deficiency as well. Over the years outbreaks of blindness have been documented from bootleg alcohol.[2] Every eye doctor is well aware that small amounts of wood alcohol are toxic to the optic nerve but are largely unaware that aspartame contains this known eye toxin.

Heavy consumers of aspartame products have been found to exceed 250 milligrams of aspartame daily, which is 32 times the limit of consumption recommended by the Environmental Protection Agency.

Here are a couple of the patient reports of eye problems related to aspartame by Dr. H.J. Roberts:

> A 36-year old woman experienced recurrent blurring of vision, unusual lights and floaters, and pain in both eyes while drinking two two-liter bottles of an aspartame orange drink.

> A 41-year old woman noted severe visual loss after drinking a diet drink. She stated: *"If I drink two or three diet colas a day I lose vision in my right eye for 10-15 minutes a session."*

Dr. Roberts had his patients stop taking aspartame and observed a cessation of their symptoms. To prove that aspartame was the true cause of their problems he had them resume taking aspartame and observed a recurrence of their eye and other health problems.

Sir Stewart Duke-Elder, the noted British ophthalmologist, lists the most common optic nerve poisons.[3] They are:

1. Tobacco (cyanide poisoning of the optic nerve)
2. Ethyl alcohol
3. Methyl alcohol, found in aspartame sweetener, or home-made brew.
4. Sedative drugs, such as barbiturates.
5. Other drugs, such as digoxin.

How many folks, who ingest foods and drinks with aspartame, also assault their optic nerve with other poisons from smoking and drugs? The combined attack of these poisons on the optic nerve should lead eye physicians to caution patients with glaucoma and other optic nerve disorders to abstain from these toxic agents.

Just as sensitive individuals may develop allergies shellfish, eggs and many other foods, some individuals may be more prone to react adversely to artificial sweeteners. It only seems wise for patients with the following ocular problems to avoid aspartame sweetened foods and drinks:

✓ Glaucoma patients
✓ Migraine or chronic headache patients
✓ Patients with dry eyes
✓ Sjogrens Syndrome patients
✓ Patients with optic neuritis
✓ Patients with any retinal disease
✓ Patients who smoke, drink or take other known eye toxins
✓ Patients with diabetic eye disease

Herbal non-caloric sugar substitute

The leaves of the stevia rebaundiana plant are the source of a non-caloric sweetener. This plant is commonly used to sweeten herb teas and is 300 times sweeter than sucrose. This natural sweetener is native to Paraguay and is used commonly in Japan, Brazil and several other countries. According to the American Herbal Products Association over 900 scientific papers substantiate the safety of stevia. Stevia leaves can be obtained from some herbal stores. Stevioside is the extracted crystalline form of this plant which can be obtained by calling B.E.D. at (404) 352-8048.

REFERENCES

[1] Sadun A.A., et al, "Epidemic optic neuropathy in Cuba," Archives of Ophthalmology 112: 691-99, 1994.
[2] Benton C.D., Calhoun F.P., "The ocular effects of methyl alcohol poisoning," American Journal of Ophthalmology, 52: 1677-85, 1952.
[3] Duke Elder E., SYSTEM OF EYE DISEASES, Volume 14, C.V. Mosby, St. Louis, p. 143-55. 1972.

Quick Facts

Part of the eye affected. *Lens, retina, eyelids, cornea, vitreous.*

Risk factors: *smoking dramatically increases the risk of cataracts, macular degeneration, diabetic retinopathy, eyelid wrinkling and many other disorders.*

Modern treatment: *smoking cessation programs. Note: blood vessels don't return to normal for 10 years following smoking cessation. Nutritional supplements are recommended to restore vascular health.*

Preventive measures: *nutritional supplements such as vitamin C, B12, folic acid, zinc, bioflavonoids.*

Questions to ask your deye octor: *Which stop-smoking programs are helpful?*

8

SMOKING AND THE EYES

Smokers may have a hunch of what this chapter is going to say--- that smoking promotes loss of vision and leads to premature development of a host of serious eye problems such as cataracts, macular degeneration and diabetic retinopathy.

Take heart. Before you become discouraged and close this section of the book you should know there are some measures to help avoid loss of vision until you can stop smoking.

A smoker cannot see the tiny blood vessels at the back of their eyes. If they could they would see that tobacco and nicotine promote the development of cyanide that destroys the optic nerve. Tobacco smoking causes the blood vessels at the back of the eye to become clogged with cholesterol and to spasm shut, robbing the ocular tissues of needed oxygen. Nicotine is known to increase blood platelet stickiness which can promote retinopathy among diabetics.[1,2]   A 5 mm rise in intraocular pressure has been demonstrated after the last puff on a cigarette.[3]

Doctors believe that the condition known as tobacco amblyopia, is rare in the U.S. and must be accompanied by alcoholism, malnutrition and vitamin B12 metabolism problems before it occurs. A recent report indicates many smokers may have mild undetected forms of optic nerve degeneration, which can develop into a visual blind spot, even though they are well nourished, do not have low levels of vitamin B12 and do not drink alcohol.[4]

Certainly smoking irritates the eyes. As smoke gets into the eyes, the eyes become red and irritated. Smokers may have no idea how

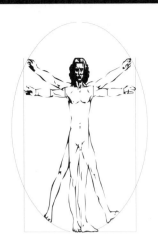

Every organ of the body is affected by tobacco smoking.

they are aging their eyes and risking their sight with every puff on a cigarette or drag on a tobacco pipe.

We now know that those individuals who smoke:

1. Develop early cataracts.

2. Subject their optic nerve to toxic levels of cyanide.

3. Suffer early onset of macular degeneration. Vision deteriorates seven years sooner at the back of the eyes of smokers.

4. Experience wrinkling and puckering of their eyelids.

5. Promote dry spots on the surface of the eyes.

Smoking tobacco inches a person towards blindness. How can this be stated in any less direct terms without scaring readers who smoke?

Smoking can aggravate glaucoma and cause it to become uncontrollable. Cataracts, which could have been stabilized with nutrition, have to be removed surgically, and macular degeneration progresses faster. Smoking re-activates herpes eye infections and exacerbates dry eyes, allergic conjunctivitis, pingueculitis, pterygia, and many other conditions.

If the smoker can get through the first two weeks without cigarettes, they will avoid the strongest withdrawal symptoms.[5] Various anti-smoking regimens are available. Discuss this topic with your physician.

There is evidence, in the face of continued smoking, that antioxidants may be helpful in minimizing the harmful effects of nicotine. Vitamin E supplements (800 units / day),[6] and N-acetyl cysteine (a glutathione precursor)[7] have been shown to be helpful.

Vitamin B12 binds with cyanide which is used in the curing of tobacco. Smokers then commonly become vitamin B12 deficient which has been linked with optic nerve degeneration. Supplementation with 500 mcgs. of vitamin B12 has been proposed for smokers as prophylaxis against optic nerve damage.[8] For every cigarette smoked the body is depleted of 25 milligrams of vitamin C.[9] A 20-cigarette per day habit means smokers need 500 milligrams of supplemental vitamin C to maintain body stores.

Smoking is known to cause premature cataracts at an annual cost of $750 million for cataract surgery. Additionally hundreds of millions of dollars are required for the treatment of diabetic eye conditions and retinal problems that are exacerbated or occur prematurely due to smoking.

REFERENCES

[1] Hawkins R.L., "Smoking, platelets and thrombosis," Nature 236: 450-52, 1972.

[2] Dobbie J.G., et al, "Role of platelets in pathogenesis of diabetic retinopathy," Archives of Ophthalmology 91: 107-09, 1974.

[3] Mehra K.S., Roy P.N., Khare B.B., "Tobacco smoking and glaucoma," Annals of Ophthalmology 8: 462-64, 1976.

[4] Rizzo J.F., Lessell S., "Tobacco amblyopia," American Journal of Ophthalmology, 116: 84-87, 1993.

[5] Wong J.G., "How to help your patients quit smoking," Postgraduate Medicine, 94: 197-98, 1993.

[6] Hoshino E., et al, "Vitamin E suppresses increased lipid peroxidation in cigarette smokers," Journal of Parenteral and Enteral Nutrition, 14: 300-05, 1990.

[7] Rogers D., et al, "Oral N-acetylcysteine speeds reversal of cigarette smoke-induced mucous cell hyperplasia in the rat," Experimental Lung Research, 14: 19-35, 1988.

[8] Kommerell G., Castrillon-Oberndorfer W.L., "Tobacco amblyopia: pathogenesis and therapy," Klin. Monatsbl. Augenheilk 153: 551-62, 1968.

[9] Pelletier O., "Vitamin C and cigarette smokers," Annals New York Academy of Sciences 258: 156-67, 1975.

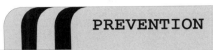

NUTRITION

PREVENTION

Summary of Preventive Measures

Until smokers can stop smoking the following list of nutritional supplements should be taken.

Vitamin C: 1000 milligrams or more daily. Slowly increase dosages of vitamin C to avoid diarrhea.

Vitamin E: 800 units daily.

N-acetyl cysteine: 100 milligrams daily.

Quercetin: 1000-3000 milligrams daily.

Vitamin B12: 500-1500 micrograms daily.

Folic acid: 400 micrograms daily.

Products by brand name that may be helpful:

Maxilife Co Q10 formula by Twinlab:
       Take 4 capsules daily

Quercetin + Vitamin C by Nature's Herbs:
       Take 2-6 capsules daily

Sublingual (under the tongue) vitamin B12:
       500-1500 micrograms per day.

Quick facts

_Part of the eye affected__: all parts of the eyes are affected by sunlight_

_Risk factors__: Ultraviolet and blue-violet sun rays. Many sunglasses in retail stores are mislabelled and give consumers a false sense of security._

_Preventive measures__: hats with 3-inch brims, total UV-blocking sun lenses, preferably with side shields._

_Questions to ask your eye doctor__:_

Do my sunglasses block all the UV rays?
Can a UV-filter be added to my prescription glasses?
How do I know if sunglasses block out all the UV rays?

9

SUNLIGHT, SUNGLASSES AND EYE HEALTH

You may already have an expensive pair of 100 percent UV-proof sunglasses. What more protection do your eyes need? If you have

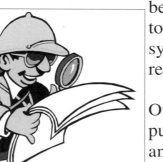

been lulled into thinking your eyes are totally protected by wearing your status-symbol sunglasses, then you need to read the rest of this chapter.

Over 100 million pair of sunglasses are purchased in the U.S. annually with total annual sales of $1.7 billion. The primary reason why people buy sunglasses is to reduce dazzling glare in bright sunlight and to make a fashion statement. One sunglass advertisement on TV showed a young man wearing his status-symbol sunglasses into a nightclub. In other words, you don't need the sun to make a fashion statement.

There is strong evidence that sunlight exposure is linked to the major eye diseases and that Americans are generally wearing the wrong kinds of sunglasses.

The problems of solar ultraviolet radiation

Imagine reading this headline in tomorrow morning's newspaper: *"Massive Radiation Leak From Power Plant; Millions Will Lose Their Eyesight."* Such a radiation leak would cause the Center for Disease Control in Atlanta to release a statement immediately warning the public to protect themselves from the radiation leak.

Because the radiation leak comes from the sun's power plant 93 million miles away and in small daily doses, it is largely overlooked by health authorities. The problem is that the populations of the world have come to associate a radiation leak with atomic energy, not the daily bombardment of invisible ultraviolet rays from the sun.

Because many believe that skin cancer is the primary threat to human health and that wearing 100 percent UV blocking sunglasses provides sufficient protection for the eyes, human populations are lulled into letting their guard down. What the public doesn't know is the sunglasses they are wearing, even the ones that have 100 percent UV filtering lenses, may actually promote a false sense of security.

Photobiologists and meteorologists warn of threats to crops, other major concerns are destruction to phytoplankton in the sea, and of skin cancer in humans. As the earth's ozone layer is gradually destroyed by man-made chemicals slowly rising into the atmosphere, *it is the human eye that is most vulnerable to damage caused by sun rays* .

An April 4, 1991 statement released by the U.S. Environmental Protection Agency warned that the depletion of the ozone layer was occurring twice as fast as predicted and that there would be a dramatic increase in the number of skin cancers over the next few decades. This statement, however, made no mention of an impending visual disaster.

An invisible hazard

The reason why UV radiation poses such a potential global health hazard is that it is imperceptible in nature. Solar ultraviolet radiation doesn't even cast a shadow, as does the visible portion of the solar spectrum. When UV rays attack the skin, pain and redness result. But when UV rays penetrate inner eye tissues (the lens and retina), there is no sensation of pain or discomfort. By the time one experiences a loss of vision it's too late to protect the eyes. Even though the UV rays pierce right through the cloud cover, humans on a cloudy day are less likely to protect their skin and

UV rays are invisible and pass through clouds

eyes. The skin does not show signs of sunburn for 6-12 hours following exposure. On overcast days the infrared heat rays are absorbed by the clouds and the skin doesn't feel as hot. The result can be an unusually severe sunburn of the skin and eyes if standing on a highly reflective surface like a snowfield or sandy beach. Elevation adds to the problem; for every 1000 feet of elevation UV radiation increases by 5 percent.

What are UV rays?

Photobiologists classify UV-B as fast tanning sun rays, while UV-A is identified as slow tanning rays. UV-B is measured as the spectrum of sunlight ranging from 280-320 nanometers on a spectrophotometer. UV-A is measured as the spectrum of sun rays between 320-400 nanometers. Currently, no sun rays below 296 nanometers reach the surface of the earth because of the protective ozone layer. With the breakdown of the ozone layer all forms of life on earth could be exposed to UV-B radiation down to 288 nanometers.[1]

Cataracts and UV rays

United Nations scientists predict an 0.6 percent increase in cataracts for every 1 percent ozone depletion. That could result in a whopping 12 percent increase in cataracts worldwide. Already cataracts blind 17 million people worldwide, and many countries do not have access to modern eye care that can replace cloudy cataracts with clear lens implants.

Chronic daily bombardment

For the most part, it is the chronic bombardment of UV rays upon the eyelids, cornea, lens, vitreous and retina that results in premature aging of the eyes, rather than a single day's exposure while sunning at the beach. Gradually, eye tissues exposed to daily UV radiation begin to break down. Proteins in the lens of the eyes begin to clump, vision becomes cloudy and cataracts form.

Sun exposure promotes the buildup of garbage deposits (called drusen) in the retina, occurring rapidly in the first three decades of life. Children's eyes are more transparent to sun rays up to age 30 when the lens of the eye develops sun-absorbing pigments resembling an internal sunglass filter for the retina. After age 50 the retina of the eye begins to lose some of its protective melanin pigment and more of these aging spots (drusen) begin to form. After six or seven decades of life this destructive process steadily destroys the light-receptor cells at the back of the eyes.

How much UV light does it take to harm the eyes?

Just a single day's exposure to the bright sun, reflected off of a snow field can result in a sunburned cornea, a condition called snow blindness (photokeratitis).

A single day's exposure to unfiltered midday sun rays on a sandy beach could result in sunburned retinas (solar retinitis) among young sunbathers. Just a few minutes of sun exposure can burn the retina, especially if there is a thinning of the earth's ozone layer.[2]

UV-B rays are generally considered more harmful to eye tissues than UV-A sun rays. UV-B rays are most intense between 10 A.M. and 2 P.M., when the sun is highest in the sky. The human eye has an elaborate natural defense against UV-B radiation. The human eye is recessed under the brow where it rests in a shadow. The lashes create an awning. The eyelids can be compressed during squinting into a narrow slit to block sun rays. The pupil of the eyes constricts, like the aperture opening in a camera, to further limit the amount of light reaching the lens and retina. The adult crystalline lens, which rests behind the pupil, turns progressively yellow throughout life and becomes an effective UV filter for the retina in most adult eyes. All of these intricate defenses are in place to protect the irreplaceable retina, the nerve center of vision. Very little UV-A and UV-B sun rays reach the retina in most adult's eyes.

The damage caused by UV radiation is cumulative; it adds up slowly over time. UV rays in large amounts reach the retina during the first thirty years of life when the eyes are more transparent and when one probably spends more time outdoors. Microscopic examination of the lens and retina of the eyes reveals that the beginnings of cataracts and retinal disease start in childhood but do not usually interfere with vision till the sixth or seventh decade of

Healthy & Hazardous:
The Good and Bad of Sun Rays

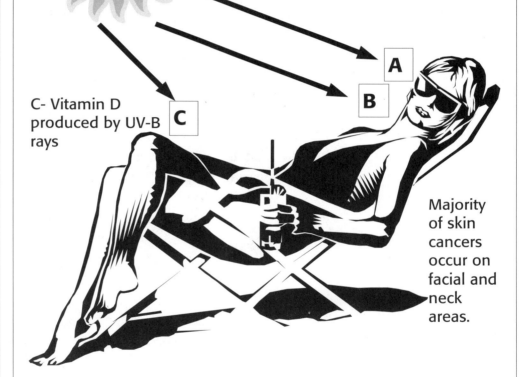

70% of UV rays reach earth's surface between 10 AM & 3 PM

A- The eyes should be protected from UV rays when outdoors, even on overcast days. No health benefits from eye exposure to UV rays.

B- UV-B rays can active Herpes lip sore

C- Vitamin D produced by UV-B rays

Majority of skin cancers occur on facial and neck areas.

UV-B sun rays produce vitamin D in the skin. Low vitamin D levels have been linked to increasesd rates of colon and breast cancer. Vitamin D is also needed to prevent osteoporosis. A few minutes of skin exposure to the sun is recommended every day. Skin damage from UV rays is cumulative over a lifetime. Too much sun increases risk of eyelid skin cancer, cataracts, pterygium and macular degeneration.

life. The importance of wearing UV-proof sunglasses and hats during the growing years cannot be overemphasized.

Most of the UV energy in adulthood is absorbed by the crystalline lens, which discolors the lens. This is why cataracts are so prevalent.

Even though very little ultraviolet radiation reaches the retina in the adult eye, Dr. Donald Pitts, optometrist and leading research scientist on the effects of UV radiation upon the human eye, indicates it only takes one photon of UV-B radiation to destroy a light-receptor cell on the retina.[3] One photon is equivalent to the light emitted by a one watt light bulb divided by one million. That's the tiniest amount of light that can be measured. While some UV-B is essential for the skin to produce vitamin D, even a little bit of UV-B radiation is harmful to the human eye.

Many adults wear semi-protective sunglasses. The tinted lenses in their sunglasses do not block out all of the UV rays. Thus the natural defense mechanisms are relaxed (squinting, aversion, pupil constriction). In a U.S. Army study, David Sliney, Ph.D., indicates it is possible for the eyes to be exposed to more UV rays when wearing partial UV protective lenses than when wearing NO sunglasses at all![4] A patrol of Marines wearing sunglasses in Greenland suffered photokeratitis (snow blindness) when wearing sunglasses that didn't block out all UV rays.[5]

Thus a tiny leak of UV-B solar radiation seeping through the ozone layer, or reaching the eyes through semi-protective sunglass lenses (bouncing into your eyes around the sides and tops of the sunglass lenses) may expose your eyes to the most harmful of all sun rays. It is these small "cracks" in our natural and artificial sun defense systems that may eventually impair sight.

How to pick the right sunglasses for your eyes

Here is a checklist of items to evaluate when purchasing a pair of sunglasses:

1. Do the lenses block out 100% of the UV-A & B? This is absolutely essential. Don't consider wearing sunglasses that permit ANY UV rays to pass through. As many as 50 million pair of

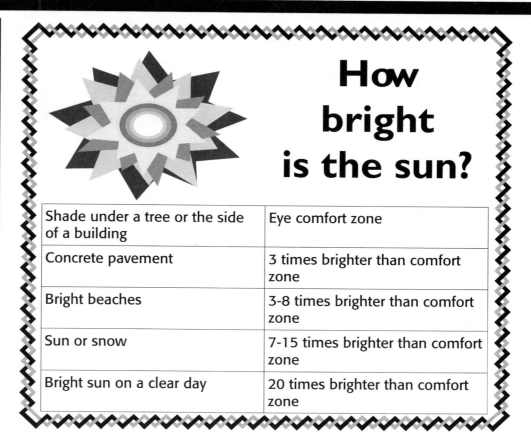

How bright is the sun?

Shade under a tree or the side of a building	Eye comfort zone
Concrete pavement	3 times brighter than comfort zone
Bright beaches	3-8 times brighter than comfort zone
Sun or snow	7-15 times brighter than comfort zone
Bright sun on a clear day	20 times brighter than comfort zone

sunglasses sold in retail stores do not provide adequate protection from UV rays.

2. How dark are the lenses? <u>The darkness of the lens has nothing to do with how much ultraviolet radiation it filters</u>. The darkest shades may cause a person to squint while wearing them. If you can't find a pair of sunglasses dark enough for eye comfort, dry eyes or other underlying eye conditions that be making the eyes extra light sensitive. If one has macular degeneration or other retinal disorders most likely a lighter tinted lens will be preferred.

3. What is the footprint of the sunglass? How large are the lenses? How much coverage do the lenses and side shields provide for your facial areas? The average size of a conventional pair of sunglasses is 40 square centimeters. For comparison, the sun coverage provided by a pair of sun goggles is 175 square centimeters, four times the protection! Sun goggles with side shields protect against airborne allergens and eye irritants, and they help to retain moisture on the surface of the eyes.

4. What material are the lenses made of? Plastic is light weight. Polycarbonate plastic is shatterproof for sports. Glass is heavier

Recommended Lens Color for Sunglasses

All sunglass lenses, regardless of color, should filter out
100 percent of UV rays (UV A & B)
Exercise caution if you have color vision problems.

VIOLET	Not recommended for macular degeneration. Alters color vision.
BLUE	Produces calming feeling; relaxing. Not recommended for macular degeneration. Recommended to reduce photosensitive epilepsy.[6,7]* (Red-free lenses) * Some epileptic seizures are provoked by light
GREEN	Best color for seasonally depressed patients.
YELLOW	Often used as shooters glasses to improve contrast. Sometimes used by cataract patients to reduce night glare. May help some macular degeneration patients during reading.
ORANGE-BROWN	UV-blue light filter; best retinal protector. Recommended for macular degeneration. Alters colors: blue and violet appear grey. 30 percent of patients may not like this lens
RED	May help patients with cone dystrophy of the retina. HAZARDOUS WHEN DRIVING; impairs colors of traffic lights.
GREY	Best for natural color perception; most popular.

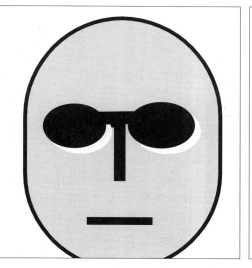
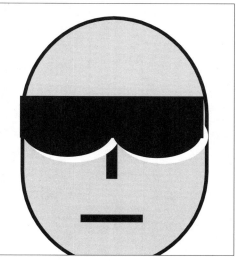

SUN COVERAGE

- ◆ Small-size sunglasses still permit peripheral sun rays to reach the eyes.

- ◆ In bright sun wearer will still squint.

- ◆ Without side shields sunglasses do not provide maximum protection against cataracts, eyelid skin cancer and pterygium

- ◆ Sun glasses or sun goggles should provide broad area of sun coverage, as shown above.

- ◆ Wrap-around design is essential- no unfiltered sun rays reach the eyes.

- ◆ Wrap-around design minimizes evaporation of tears.

but can contain a polarized film to reduce reflected glare.

5. How durable is the sunglass product? If lenses can pop out of the frames easily the glasses may not last.

6. If prescription eyeglasses are worn one can purchase wrap-around goggles that fit over glasses and save on the cost of a pair of prescription sunglasses (savings of about $170 savings).

7. Surveys of sunglasses on store displays reveal that as much as 40 percent of sunglass products are mislabelled.[8] Even some UV protective coatings applied by opticians on prescription eyeglasses have been found to be deficient in blocking UV rays.[9] The Food &

Drug Administration is developing updated codes for sunglass labelling.

How can consumers check up on false labelling? Obtain an ULTRAVIOLET SENSOMETER made by Optiwear, a wallet-card size UV sensor. Light-sensitive chemicals in the card turn color when exposed to UV sun rays. By placing the sunglasses over the card you can tell if the lenses block out all UV rays. The ULTRAVIOLET SENSOMETER is available for $5 from Optiwear, 3100 James Street, Syracuse, NY 13206.

8. Are the lenses scratch-protected? If they are, they won't scratch as easily when you clean them.

9. What's the best color of sunglass lens? Grey and green lenses are the most popular and produce the most natural view.

10. What about the blue-filter lenses? The retina of the human eye is sensitive to damage from UV and blue-violet sun rays. For this reason many people are advised to wear UV-blue violet filtering lenses, which appear brown in color. These blue filter lenses enhance depth perception, but they do alter color perception. The blue sky appears grey. People with retinal disorders who have blue eyes and are exposed to a lot of midday sun rays, might want to try on a pair of these lenses. Up to a third of people who try these blue stopping lenses don't like them and pick a grey lens instead.[10]

11. If cataracts have been removed UV-filtering sunglasses need to be worn. Most lens implants inside the eyes have built-in chemical UV filters, but they may not block out all of the UV rays and they still do not protect the retina from blue-violet radiation, nor the cornea and eyelids.

12. Polarized lenses are popular and work best when driving on a flat road or fishing on a calm body of water. Polarization doesn't have anything to do with UV protection.

13. Mirrored or glass sunglass lenses help to block out infrared heat rays. Infrared filters help to cool the eyes.

14. The best combination of eye protection is a hat and sunglasses. Hats should have three inch brims to fully cover facial areas in

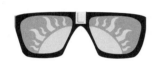

For a free list of UV-blocking sunglasses by brand name write to:

Richard W. Young, Ph.D.
UCLA Medical School
Los Angeles, California 90024-1763

shade.

15. There is a condition known as Seasonal Affective Disorder. This condition causes depression, carbohydrate craving and sleep disorder and is often found among adults who live in less-sunny northern areas. Bright sunlight or artificial light can help to reduce symptoms of depression by stimulating the optic nerve, which in turn stimulates the pineal gland at the base of the brain. Visible light rays (not the invisible UV rays) produce the health benefits for individuals who are seasonally depressed. During winter months, depressed persons should avoid habitual wearing of darkly tinted lenses. Clear prescription lenses with 100 percent UV filters are suggested.

16. An estimated 6 percent of skin cancers occur around the eye lids.[11] Only wrap-around sun lenses will provide complete UV protection for the eyelids.

17. One research study has demonstrated how sun rays reaching the eyes from the side, around conventional sunglass lenses, can produce abnormal growths on the surface of the eyes (pterygium) and cortical cataracts.[12] Conventional sunglasses without side or top shields have been shown to permit as much as 45 percent of the sun rays to reach the eyes.[13]   To repeat: if your sunglasses don't have side shields, your eyes aren't totally protected from UV sun rays.

18. Cheap children's sunglasses, often sold in toy stores, are often mislabelled and have been shown to be a potential hazard to children's eyes.[14] Children should be taught the habit of wearing UV protective sunglasses and hats in bright sun. For a catalog of 100 percent UV-protective sunglasses for children and other sun-protection gear write to Sun Precautions, 168 Denny Way, Seattle, Washington 98109.

For a minimal investment, and no side effects, anyone can take advantage of the preventive benefits offered by a good pair of sunglasses.

REFERENCES

[1] Pitts, D., "Sunlight as an ultraviolet source," Optometry & Vision Science, 67: 401-06, 1990.

[2] Yannuzzi L.A., Fisher Y.L., Slakter J.S., Krueger A., "Solar Retinopathy," Retina, 9: 28-43, 1989.

[3] Pitts D.G., "Ultraviolet-absorbing spectacle lenses, contact lenses, and intraocular lenses," Optometry and Vision Science 67: 435-40, 1990.

[4] Sliney D.H., "Eye protective techniques for bright light," Ophthalmology, 90: 937-44, 1983.

[5] Correspondence from David H. Sliney, Ph.D., February 1, 1993.

[6] Takahashi T., Tsukahara Y., "Usefulness of blue sunglasses in photosensitive epilepsy," Epilepsia, 33: 517-21, 1992.

[7] Newmark M.E., Penry J.K., PHOTOSENSITIVE EPILEPSY: A REVIEW, Raven Press, New York, 1987, pp. 9-11 and 128-29.

[8] Thomas, S.R., "Comparison of radiometric transmittance properties of sunglasses to ANSI Z80.3 (1986) standards," Poster, American Academy of Optometry, December, 1991.

[9] van Kuijk F., "Effects of ultraviolet light on the eye: role of protective glasses," Environmental Health Perspectives, 96: 177-84, 1991.

[10] Pitts D.G., Kleinstein R.N., ENVIRONMENTAL VISION, Butterworth-Heinemann, London, 1993, p. 309.

[11] Suarez-Varela M.M., Gonzalez A.L., Caraco E.F., "Non-melanoma skin cancer: an evaluation of risk in terms of ultraviolet exposure," European Journal of Epidemiology, 8: 838-44, 1992.

[12] Coroneo M.T., Muller-Stolzenburg N.W., Ho A., "Peripheral light focusing by the anterior eye and the ophthalmohelioses," Ophthalmic Surgery, 22: 705-11, 1991.

[13] Rosenthal F.S., Bakalian A.E., Lou C., Taylor H.R., "The effect of sunglasses on ocular exposure to ultraviolet radiation," American Journal of Public Health, 78: 72-74, 1988.

[14] Werner J.S., "Children's sunglasses: caveat emptor," Optometry & Vision Sciences, 88: 318-20, 1991.

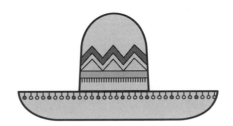

Low-Technology Sun Protection

A hat with a three-inch brim affords protection for sensitive eye and facial areas where skin cancers often develop.

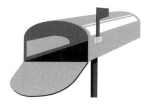

Mail bag

I'm writing for my husband since his vision is very bad and it is difficult for him to write. Ten years ago coumadin (a blood-thinning drug) caused a bleeding in the visual center of the brain and that took away 50 percent of his sight in his right eye. Is there anything that can be done?

J.S.
Pompano Beach, Florida

10
SIDE EFFECTS OF DRUGS

Of the 20 most prescribed drugs, 10 can cause blurred or distorted vision and 9 are reported to cause dry eyes.[1]

Many commonly used medications can produce ocular side effects. Additionally, many eye drops and medications used for eye conditions have side effects on the rest of the body. Most intriguing is the relationship between sunlight and drugs within the human eye. Many seemingly mysterious eye disorders originate from side effects produced by drugs.

[The major sources for the following information are the PHYSICIAN'S DESK REFERENCE FOR OPHTHALMOLOGY (Weisbecker C.A., Naidoff M., Tippermann R., Medical Economics, Montvale, NJ., 1993] and; DRUG-INDUCED OCULAR SIDE EFFECTS AND DRUG INTERACTIONS, F.T. Fraunfelder, Meyer S.M., 2nd edition, Lea & Febiger, Philadelphia, 1982.

Drugs that cause eye problems

Cocaine

There is growing concern over the number of young adults who are chronic cocaine users and who come to the ophthalmologist's office with serious eye infections, some resulting in corneal ulcers and scarred corneas with loss of vision.[2] Organisms like Staphylococcus, Streptococcus and Candida are found growing on the surface of the corneas of crack cocaine abusers.

Cocaine is an eye anesthetic, one of the first to be used on the eyes. The cocaine numbs the cornea, and the individual doesn't blink as

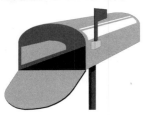

I have this problem with imbalance which I believe is from these medications--- the side effects are weak muscles. The doctors don't say so but the information on them does say so. I am hoping you can recommend something else for treatment minus these side effects.

S.M.
Central Valley,
California

often. Eventually unwanted organisms grow on the surface of the eyes. The outer layer of the cornea (epithelium) breaks down, giving organisms a chance to grow.[3] Cocaine users are generally unaware they could lose their sight by chronic use of this drug.

Retina-A

Retin-A (isotretinoin) is a popularly used topical medication for skin aging and acne. Oral administration of this medication has resulted in eye inflammation, dry eyes, contact lens intolerance and corneal opacities. The topical form used by dermatologists may cause poor night vision, excessive glare sensitivity, and abnormal retinal function. Because this medication has been shown to mimic the same retinal changes observed in "hereditary" retinal disorders such as retinitis pigmentosa (RP), researchers recommend that its use among RP patients or family members be avoided.[4] Dermatologists should recommend that their Retin-A patients wear UV-protective sun goggles. **Exposure to bright sunlight should be avoided during Retin-A therapy.** Also avoid use in cases of optic neuritis.

Diazepam (Valium)

This popularly used relaxant has been reported to cause allergic conjunctivitis (red eye), involuntary eye twitching, and some paralysis of eye muscles. Users should be aware of ocular side effects.

Oral contraceptives

Women with visual disturbances using birth control pills or hormones for the change of life should undergo a medical eye examination by an ophthalmologist. Oral contraceptive users have a higher incidence of migraine headaches, blood clotting disorders, difficulties wearing contact lenses, and with long-term use color vision abnormalities. Avoid use of birth control pills or hormones if there are known retinal disorders or ophthalmic migraines.

There is no "safe" dosage for steroid eye drops.

Steroids (corticosteroids)

Steroidal preparations are made to replace hormones produced by the adrenal glands and are used to help reduce inflammation or allergy reactions. **Ocular side effects from the use of steroids probably cause the most numerous eye problems because they are so commonly used.** Steroids cause cataracts, glaucoma, subconjunctival hemorrhages, myopia and many other eye problems. As patients have individual sensitivity, there is no "safe" eye drop dosage for steroids. Ocular side effects from steroid eye drops may take a while before they become apparent. One study showed that half of the patients who administered 800 drops of a steroid eye drop developed some early-stage cataracts. **The cataract-causing effects of steroid eye drops may be counteracted by taking high dosages of vitamin C, E, and other antioxidants.** Most steroid-induced glaucomas are reversible.

Glaucoma drops

Glaucoma patients should not be so overly concerned about the side effects from glaucoma medications that they avoid taking the medication. Glaucoma patients should be aware, however, that the most popularly used glaucoma eye drops (beta blockers such as TImolol, Timoptic, Betagan) may produce side effects such as fatigue, depression, and loss of libido. Because beta blocker drugs may exacerbate asthma they should not be taken by individuals who have breathing problems.

Digoxin: Used for heart failure or heart irregularity

Color vision changes, especially yellow colorations, and snowy appearance of objects are the most common side effects from taking digitalis drugs; light flashes, blind spots and aversion to light are other reported symptoms. As many as one in four heart patients taking digitalis report eye side effects.

Blood pressure medications and low-pressure glaucoma

Approximately 10 percent of glaucoma patients have what is called "low-pressure" glaucoma. The fluid pressure with this type of glaucoma is normal or below normal but the optic nerve at the back of the eye is still damaged. This in contrary to the common form of glaucoma where high fluid pressure damages the optic nerves at the back of the eyes. General practitioners often advise their patients to take blood pressure lowering drugs at bedtime to minimize any side effects during waking hours, such as dizziness. However blood pressure lowering drugs taken at bedtime may reduce eye fluid pressure too much and may aggravate this type of glaucoma.[5]

Sjogrens Syndrome

Arthritic patients may suffer with dry eyes and/or Sjogrens' Syndrome (dry eye and dry mouth). One particular anti-arthritic drug, Levamisol, may actually increase dry eye problems and should be avoided if the patient has a pre-existing dry eye. Chemotherapy drugs for treatment of cancer also commonly produce dry eye symptoms.

Aspartame (Nutrasweet)

The artificial sweetener aspartame (Nutrasweet, Searle Pharmaceuticals) has been associated with numerous ocular side effects.

This product is the combination of two amino acids: L-aspartic acid and L-phenylalanine. While the Council on Scientific Affairs has concluded that aspartame is safe, there may be individuals who are sensitive to this sweetener. This is especially true of those who consume significant amounts in diet drinks, as a sweetener in their coffee, chewing gum, etc.

One in 15,000 people in this country, about 17,000 Americans, have a condition known as phenylketonuria (PKU) where they lack the enzyme to metabolize phenylalanine (an amino acid found in aspartame). These PKU patients may experience dizziness, headache, and sleeping problems when taking aspartame. Individuals who do not have PKU may also not be able to tolerate elevated levels of phenylalanine and exhibit the same symptoms. Aspartame is not "totally" safe for every individual.

Among patients who have the Sjogrens Syndrome form of dry eyes, it has been shown that aspartame also promotes dry mouth and creates a vicious thirst for more aspartame-containing drinks to moisten their mouths. Aspartame has been shown to exacerbate contact lens intolerance among dry eyed individuals.[6]

The greatest concern over the use of aspartame among eye doctors is its chemical similarity to methyl alcohol. Raw wood alcohol (methanol or methyl alcohol), which is known to be a retinal toxic agent in moonshine whiskey, can destroy the optic nerve.

Bootleg whiskey that contained 35 percent methyl alcohol and 15 percent ethyl alcohol ended up killing 37 of 320 patients who drank the illegal brew. Within 18-48 hours of ingestion, many other users began seeing spots before their eyes and some reported complete blindness.[7]

Is a small amount of aspartame found in diet drinks and coffee sweeteners capable of adversely affecting the optic nerve of the human eye? Some sensitive adults whose intake of aspartame is high have developed transient and permanent loss of vision. While there may be debate over whether aspartame sweetener could contribute to eye problems, there is little doubt that some eye problems disappear when a person stops taking aspartame. Any patients who have dry eyes, migraine headaches, vitreous floaters, optic nerve disorders (glaucoma, optic neuritis) or retinal problems such as retinitis pigmentosa or macular degeneration, should stop using aspartame-containing foods and sweeteners.

While aspartame is 200 times sweeter than sugar, the annual per capita consumption of sugar has not been reduced since the introduction of artificial sweeteners. An estimated 54 percent of Americans use aspartame products.

Photosensitive drugs

The list of drugs that increase sensitivity to sunlight is lengthy. Six of the 20 most prescribed drugs increase sensitivity to the sun. The Food & Drug Administration has issued a list of many of these photosensitizing drugs.[8] Photosensitizing drugs are truly dangerous to sight 100 percent if UV--protective eye wear is not worn. Some of them are:

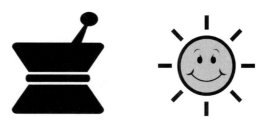

Drugs that don't mix with the sun

- Antihistamines
- Coal tar preparations for skin and scalp conditions
- Oral contraceptives
- Anti-arthritic drugs (Ibuprofen, Indomethacin, Naproxen, Sulindac)
- Tranquilizers (Thioridazine, Chlorpromazine)
- Sulfa drugs
- Oral anti-diabetic drugs (Diabinase, Orinase)
- Water pills to reduce blood pressure (Hydrochlorothiazide, furosemide, Lasix)
- Tetracycline antibiotics (Tetracycline, Doxycycline, Vibramycin)
- Anti-depressants (Amitriptyline, Elavil)
- Acetazolamide anti-glaucoma medication (Diamox)
- Diclofenac (Voltaren eye drop)
- Hexachlorophene (Phisohex) antibacterial cleanser
- Hydrochlorothiazide (Hydrodiuril, Dyazide) blood pressure lowering drug
- Ibuprofen (Advil, Motrin)
- Minoxidol (Rogaine) for baldness
- Naprosyn (Anaprox) for arthritis
- Procardia (Nifedipine) for angina
- Phenergan antihistamine
- Reserpine (Ser-Ap-Es) blood pressure drug
- Sulindac (Clinoril) for arthritis
- Bactrim urinary tract antibiotic
- Timolol + hydrochlorothiazide glaucoma eye drop + blood pressure drug

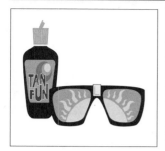

When taking photo-sensitizing medications sunglasses and sunscreens are suggested when outdoors in bright sun.

Pharmacists often affix a label indicating many of these drugs are sun sensitive, but many times this is overlooked.

Certain photosensitizing drugs make it easier for ultraviolet sun rays to cause problems within the eyes. **Over 180 different drugs can cause a photosensitive reaction in the eyes.**

Many senior Americans undergo cataract operations which increase the amount of sunlight reaching the retina. Many individuals are also taking water pills (hydrochlorothiazide diuretics) which can damage the retina in combination with UV sun rays. Most of these drugs are activated by both UV-A & B sun rays.[9] Anyone taking them for a long period of time, or anyone exposed to bright sunlight while taking these medications -- especially following cataract removal, should wear wrap-around 100 percent UV filtering sun goggles.

Patients undergoing (bright light) phototherapy for depression should be carefully screened to determine if they take any photosensitizing anti-depressant drugs.[10]

The medication <u>allopurinol</u> (Zyloprim, Lopurin) used to treat gout may produce cataracts after two years of use, especially among people who live in sunny areas. Researchers have recommended UV sun protection for patients with gout taking this medicine.[11]

<u>Epinephrine</u> eye drops are used to treat the most common form of glaucoma. These drops decrease the production of fluid within the eyes and they also constrict blood vessels and widen the pupil. Epinephrine turns brown when exposed to sunlight, and it will discolor contact lenses with continued use in sunlight. Patients who have had cataracts removed and are prescribed epinephrine should wear total UV-protective sun goggles. Not all cataract lens implants block out the entire spectrum of UV sun rays.

<u>Oxsoralen</u> (methoxsalen), a drug used to treat skin conditions like psoriasis and vitiligo in combination with UV radiation, is known to cause cataracts. The photosensitizing drug gets into the natural lens of the eye where it is chemically bound and can eventually discolor the lens, resulting in a cataract. This should not deter patients from undergoing treatment for psoriasis, but patients must be warned to wear total UV-protective lenses for 24 hours

following drug ingestion.   Even the light from fluorescent lamps can cause this reaction so UV-tinted lenses should be worn indoors as well.[12]

Plaquenil and chloroquine, antimalarial drugs, are also known to cause corneal and retinal problems. These drugs are often used to treat collagen diseases such as lupus and various forms of arthritis.

REFERENCES

[1] Pamphlet, SIDE EFFECTS OF THE 20 MOST PRESCRIBED DRUGS, H.R. Pilelsky Inc.
[2] Sachs R., et al, "Corneal complications associated with the use of crack cocaine," Ophthalmology 100: 187-91, 1993.
[3] Hersh P.S., "Use of crack cocaine tied to corneal damage," Ophthalmology Times, February 15, 1992, p. 13.
[4] Feist R.M., Kimble J.A., Morris R.E., Witherspoon C.D., "Visual side effects of isotretinoin therapy," Southern Medical Journal, 80: `332, 1987.
[5] Siegel, L., "Taking blood pressure medicine at bedtime seen as eyesight risk," Associated Press, September 1992, at the Research to Prevent Blindness Science Writers Seminar.
[6] Roberts H.J., "Aspartame-Associated Dry Mouth (Xerostomia)," Townsend Letter for Doctors, March, 1993, pp. 201-02.
[7] Benton C.D., Calhoun F.P., Jr., "The ocular effects of methyl alcohol poisoning: report of a catastrophe involving 320 persons," American Journal of Ophthalmology, 36: 1677-85, 1953.
[8]Levine J.I., MEDICATIONS THAT INCREASE SENSITIVITY TO LIGHT: A 1990 LISTING, HHS Publication FDA 91-8280, December 1990.
[9] Robert J.E., Reme C.E., Dillon J., Terman M., "Exposure to bright light and the concurrent use of photosensitizing drugs," The New England Journal of Medicine, May 28, 1992, p. 1500-01.
[10] Whitt R., Darzy S., Dillon J., Roberts J.E., "Potential phototoxicity of antidepressant drugs," Investigative Ophthalmology, 16: ARVO Abstracts, March 15, 1991.
[11] Fraunfelder F., Lerman S., "Allopurinol therapy (letter)," American Journal of Ophthalmology, 99: 215-16, 1985.
[12] Lerman S., "Light-induced changes in ocular tissues," in CLINICAL LIGHT DAMAGE TO THE EYE, D. Miller, editor, Spring-Verlag, New York, 1987, pp. 183-215.

Quick facts

Part of the eye affected: whole eye

Risk factors: yeast overgrowth in the digestive tract; lack of digestive juices

Modern treatment: Prescription medications

Preventive measures: High fiber diets, yogurt or acdiophilus/bifidus supplements; bottled water in lieu of tap water; herbs to control yeast.

Questions to ask your doctor:

Are there any nutritional ways of controlling digestive diseases?

11

EYE PROBLEMS AND DIGESTIVE DISORDERS

Older adults are ten times more likely to experience eye disorders. When taking a medical history from adults who have cataracts, macular degeneration, or a host of other eye disorders, many often report they have digestive tract problems. Included here are problems such as irritable bowel, ulcerative colitis (Crohn's disease), pancreatitis, liver troubles, and just plain indigestion and gas and bloating after meals. Many people with eye problems have trouble just taking a vitamin pill, mostly because of a lack of digestive juices in their stomach.

Eye problems have been linked to malabsorption of various nutrients caused by an unhealthy digestive tract. Here is a list of some of them:

⇒ As has been discussed earlier in this book, the lack of absorption of thiamine (vitamin B1) has been linked with the occurrence of glaucoma.[1]

⇒ A lack of digestive juices (hydrochloric acid) has been shown to cause a riboflavin deficiency that results in ocular rosacea (red irritated eyes and red cheeks).[2]

⇒ Digestive malabsorption syndrome or chronic liver disease may result in night vision problems.[3]

⇒ Individuals who have the Sjogrens syndrome variety of dry eyes, with accompanying dry mouth and arthritis, have been shown to have very low levels of digestive juices. These lead to symptoms of fatigue and allergy sensitivity.[4]

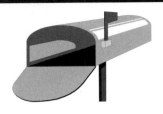

Mail bag

I have floaters and the gel behind my eye is drying up. My eye doctor said we don't know what causes it. He gave me eye drops. Is beta carotene good for the eyes? I have ulcerative colitis. This eye was blind years ago, then it got cured. The only thing the doctor surmised something could have got in the blood stream from the colitis.

L.D.
Limestone, Maine

⇒ An estimated 30 percent of uveitis patients exhibit overgrowth of pathogenic bacteria in the bowels.[5]

⇒ Progressive (pathologic) myopia, a condition that usually occurs between the ages of 40 and 60, affects 6-18 percent of all nearsighted adults. Some researchers have suggested that problems with fat absorption may be involved in this eye problem and that supplementary doses of fatty vitamins A and E should be considered.[6]

⇒ In some people, if the good bacteria that controls the overgrowth of yeast in the digestive tract are destroyed by antibiotics, yeast is left to grow unchecked. Yeast in the digestive tract "craves" sugars, which may then lead to blood sugar problems and accompanying eye problems.

The fact that eye problems are prevalent among the population of senior Americans, and digestive problems are common among the elderly, should cause further investigation of the link between digestive disorders and vision.

Following is a list of digestive tract disorders, that may be caused by vitamin deficiencies, and could result in eye problems.

Liver disease

Degenerative liver disease can result in progressive decay of the cone cells (color vision cells) of the retina.[7] Patients with liver disease, for example cirrhosis from alcoholism, may experience diminished night vision and drying of the surface of the eyes.

Fat malabsorption leads to a lack of vitamin A, a fatty vitamin. Vitamin A absorption is enhanced by bile, which is impaired in liver disease.[8]

The body makes its own natural antioxidants, such as glutathione, catalase, super oxide dismutase and coenzyme Q10. The liver is also the storehouse of these antioxidants, which are known to protect all parts of the human eye from disease. A healthy liver is important to remain free of disease, especially eye disease.

In traditional Chinese medicine doctors treat inflammation in the eye in the same manner they treat constipation. These healers know there is a link between the digestive tract and ocular health.

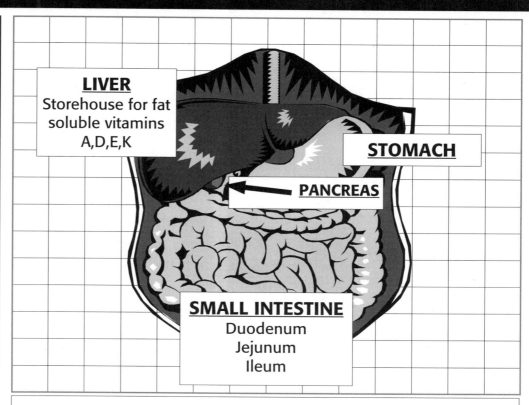

LIVER
Storehouse for fat soluble vitamins A,D,E,K

STOMACH

PANCREAS

SMALL INTESTINE
Duodenum
Jejunum
Ileum

DIGESTIVE TRACT

DIGESTIVE JUICES ARE NECESSARY TO ABSORB NUTRIENTS

Bile	Necessary for absorption of vitamin E	Liver
Insulin	Secrete insulin for metabolism of sugars	Pancreas
Amylase	Digests starches	Pancreas
Protease	Digests proteins	Pancreas
Lipase	Digests fats	Pancreas
Pepsin	Helps digest amino acids (Tyrosine, tryptophan, phenylalanine)	Pancreas
Hydrochloric acid	Digests zinc, calcium, vitamin C, B-vitamins, many others	Digestive tract

Zinc, copper and selenium are normally excreted in the bile and reabsorbed by the intestine. But when bowel function is abnormal, their reabsorption is limited. Deficiencies that affect vision can result.

Crohn's disease and ulcerative colitis

Approximately 10 percent of patients with Crohn's disease experience eye problems related to their digestive tract problems.[9] Diarrhea is a chronic problem for these patients. Diarrhea often leads to loss of electrolytes such as potassium, magnesium, and sodium, and inhibits the reabsorption of vitamins A, D, and E. Again, these are nutrients important to the eyes. Prolonged diarrhea (gastroenteritis) has been linked with cataracts, corneal problems and the formation of Bitot's spots among malnourished children in third world countries.[10]

The most common eye symptom of Crohn's Disease is inflammation of the sclera, white of the eyes, which can be painful. This can result in light sensitivity, inflammation inside the eyes (uveitis, iritis), corneal opacities, and retinal swelling. Vitamin A deficiency may result in night blindness and dry eyes (reduced mucin production).

Crohn's disease patients often have poor vitamin A absorption. Crohn's patients who were underweight, had poor vitamin A levels and exhibited symptoms of night blindness.[11] These patients also become zinc deficient and develop impaired night vision, which can be improved with zinc supplementation.[12]

Crohn's disease, or ulcerative colitis, is associated with poor absorption of nutrients from foods, including B12, folic acid, vitamin A, zinc, C, E, selenium, and magnesium.[13]

An estimated 50-100,000 new cases of irritable bowel disease and Crohn's disease are newly diagnosed each year in the U.S., mostly among adults aged 15-35.

A multivitamin formula along with additional magnesium (600 milligrams), zinc (up to 30 milligrams), vitamin A and vitamin E

Few would argue that vitamins are not essential for ocular health. For example, vitamin A for maintenance of night vision and mucin production in the tear film. However, nutrients must be digested properly before they can be utilized by the eye.

has been advocated for adults with these digestive tract disorders.[14] The diet should consist of fish, rice, oats and vegetables, along with vitamin supplements, digestive enzymes, and acidophilus/bifidus bacteria (yogurt culture).

Pancreatitis

Pancreatitis, often caused by alcoholism or gallstones, may lead to destruction of the insulin producing cells and to diabetes. Due to a lack of oxygen reaching the retina, pancreatitis may lead to a sudden loss of vision.[15]

Parasites and bacteria

The elderly digestive tract, and those who have compromised immune systems as the elderly often do, may have any number of parasites, bacterium or virus in their gastrointestinal tract. These include Giardia lamblia, Shigella, Salmonella, Campylobacter, amoeba, Herpes Simplex, cytomegalovirus, and others.[16] The toxins emanating from these foreign growths may interfere with normal nutrition needed for eye health.

Hydrochloric acid deficiency

The prevalence of atrophic gastritis, lack of digestive acid, ranges from 24 percent to 37 percent among adults aged 60-80. Some nutritional experts estimated 50% of older adults have this problem.[17]

A lack of digestive juices has been linked with malabsorption of vitamin C and numerous B vitamins, as well as many minerals. Vitamin deficiencies from malabsorption have been linked with various eye disorders.[18]

B vitamins, which have been shown to be poorly absorbed in the digestive tract without adequate levels of hydrochloric acid, may be involved in retinal diseases. Animal studies have shown that deficiencies of B vitamins can lead to deterioration of the retina and choroid layers at the back of the eyes.[19]

When the gastric tract produces an insufficient amount of stomach

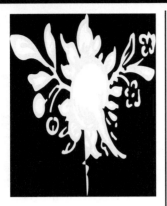

Flowering Garlic

acid (hydrochloric acid), a deficiency of an enzyme needed for absorption of vitamin B12 may result. The condition is called pernicious anemia and can result in shrinkage of the optic nerve. Men who smoke comprise the majority of these cases of optic nerve deterioration.[20]

Yeast overgrowth (thrush/candida)

When hydrochloric acid is lacking in the digestive tract, yeast growth is uncontrolled. The factors which predispose to chronic intestinal overgrowth of yeast, also called thrush or candida, are:

1. Recurrent or prolonged treatment with antibiotics
2. Prolonged use of the contraceptive pill
3. Prolonged treatment with cortisone
4. Multiple pregnancies
5. A history of high sugar consumption
6. Ingestion of large quantities of yeast products (alcohol, cheeses, mushrooms)

The overgrowth of yeast in the digestive tract may produce the following symptoms:

- ○ Bloating and gas
- ○ Chronic rectal irritation
- ○ Chronic vaginal yeast infections
- ○ Cystitis (bladder infections)
- ○ Depression, irritability
- ○ Nervous indigestion (often misdiagnosed as hiatal hernia)
- ○ Chronic constipation
- ○ Fungal rashes on the body, under nails[21]

Garlic helps to retard the overgrowth of yeast in the digestive tract and helps to destroy "bad" bacteria, viruses and parasites. Odorless garlic may have no effect.[22]

Vitamin deficiencies are common among the elderly

Vitamin deficiencies may not be easily detected in the elderly. **Up to 56 percent of the elderly are deficient in one or more**

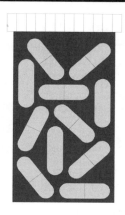

When nutrients cannot be obtained or digested from foods, vitamin supplements may be required for health maintenance

vitamins and even after supplementation in up to 39 percent of cases.[23]

Studies reveal that 42-65 percent of the elderly don't get enough Vitamin A in their diet. Vitamin A is an important vitamin for the health of the retina, cornea, and lens, and is given as a treatment for diminished night vision. Diuretics, often prescribed for blood pressure control among senior Americans, can cause loss of magnesium, potassium and zinc, exacerbating nutritional deficiencies.

Over time, poor intake of vitamins by the elderly, along with poor absorption of nutrients, may result in various health problems including eye disorders.

It is difficult to prove that digestive disorders contribute to eye problems in a particular patient. Family doctors and internists are likely to dismiss eye problems as being separate from digestive problems.

Promoting digestive tract health

The intestinal flora of an individual is composed of 100 trillion viable bacteria, representing more than 100 different types of bacterial species. The digestive tract should be replenished with a fresh supply of "good bacteria" on a regular basis. **This involves supplements with acidophilus and bifidus bacteria, preferably taken with spring water which has the correct pH so that "good" bacteria will thrive.** High fiber diets have been shown to enhance the balance of good intestinal bacteria. Nutritional scientists have shown that the bifidobacterium is probably the most important of all the bacteria needed in the digestive tract, more so than acidophilus. **A popular Chinese herb, panax ginseng, has been shown to enhance the growth of good bacteria in the gastric tract.**[24]

Note: Do not take acidophilus supplements with tap water, since it contains chlorine that may kill the good bacteria. Chlorine in tap water could be a major reason why the American digestive tract ages prematurely.

Digestive enzymes derived from plants, such as papaya enzyme, may be taken safely. Other digestive enzymes hydrochloric acid, pancreatin, pepsin and bile, should be taken under the advice and watchful eye of a physician. Do not take hydrochloric acid supplements if you have ulcers, hiatal hernia or taking antiinflammatory drugs. Consult with your physician. Bromelain (pineapple enzyme) and papain (papaya enzyme) are easily tolerated digestive aids and can be acquired in most health food stores.

Taking a little apple cider vinegar just prior to eating can naturally stimulate the production of digestive juices. Cayenne pepper has a similar action.

Antacids and nutrition

Antacids are commonly touted because they contain calcium required for strong bones among aging women who commonly develop brittle bones in later life. Antacids neutralize stomach acid upon which the absorption of many nutrients, including calcium, magnesium, zinc, vitamin C, and many others is dependant. Taking any antacid regularly will cause the body to become undernourished.[25] Anyone with an eye disease should be discouraged from taking antacids.

It is obvious from the discussion above that nutritional supplements taken for eye conditions may be poorly absorbed unless digestive problems are overcome.

Herbs to improve digestion

There are various natural herbs that can be taken as mild digestive aids.[26] Some of these are:

⚙ Apple cider vinegar. A teaspoon taken prior to a meal helps stimulate digestive juices.

⚙Fennel seed. Relaxes spasm of smooth muscles in the stomach and relieves gas

⚙Cinnamon. Aids in the digestion of fats; fights yeast

❁ <u>Ginger</u>. Relaxes spasm of smooth muscles in the stomach and relieves gas

❁ <u>Peppermint</u>. Stimulates bile; soothes digestive tract

❁ <u>Papaya</u>. Contains papain whose enzymes are similar to pepsin produced in the digestive tract; helps to digest proteins, starches and milk proteins.

❁ <u>Red (cayenne) pepper</u>. Stimulates the production of digestive juices.

❁ <u>Rosemary</u>. Relaxes smooth muscles in the stomach.

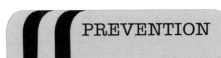

NUTRITION   **PREVENTION**

Summary program to preserve digestive tract health.

1. Eat high fiber foods daily. Persons with irritable bowel or chronic diarrhea may need to consult with a physician before increasing fiber.

2. Eat yogurt with active cultures of Bifidus or Lactobacillus weekly. Or take cultured supplements with spring water. Take yogurt culures in between courses of antibiotics. Drink bottled water instead of tap water to avoid chlorine.

3. Watch for signs of yeast overgrowth in the digestive tract such as bloating, air, gas, sugar craving, coated tongue, fatigue. Herbs like garlic, cinnamon and ginseng help to keep yeast growth in check.

4. To aid in digestion, eat fresh raw (uncooked) fruits and vegetables which have their own digestive juices.

5. Avoid chronic use of antacids and eat acid foods that aid digestion.

6. Supplement with digestive enzymes under the watchful supervision of your physician. Hydrochloric acid supplements should not be taken if there is a hiatal hernia, ulcers or taking anti-inflammatory drugs.

7. Don't ignore signs such as chronic diarrhea, constipation, indigestion.

REFERENCES

[1] Asregadoo E.R., "Blood levels of thiamine and ascorbic acid in chronic open angle glaucoma," Annals of Ophthalmology 11: 1095-1100, 1979.

[2] Johnson L.V., Eckardt R.E., "Rosacea keratitis and conditions with vascularization of cornea treated with riboflavin," Archives of Ophthalmology, 23: 899-907, 1940.

[3] Newsome D.A., "Laboratory and diagnostic studies as adjuncts to the evaluation of retinal dystrophies and degenerations," in RETINAL DYSTROPHIES AND DEGENERATIONS, D.A. Newsome, editor, Raven Press, New York, 1988, p. 73.

[4] Maury C.P.J., Tornroth T., Teppo A.M., "Atrophic gastritis in Sjogens Syndrome," Arthritis and Rheumatism, 28: 389-94, 1985.

[5] Trew D., "Bowel flora may be linked to acute anterior uveitis cases," Ophthalmology Times, September 1, 1990, p. 11.

[6] Blacharski P.A., "Pathologic progressive myopia," in RETINAL DYSTROPHIES AND DEGENERATIONS, D.A. Newsome, editor, Raven Press, New York, 1988.

[7] Berg K., Larsen I.F., Hansen, E., "Familial syndrome of progressive cone dystrophy, degenerative liver disease, and endocrine dysfunction, III genetic studies," Clinical Genetics, 13: 190-200, 1978.

[8] Romanchuk K.G., "Hepatic disease," in THE EYE IN SYSTEMIC DISEASE, D.H. Gold, T.A. Weingeist, editor, J. B. Lippincott, Philadelphia, 1990, pp. 101-02.

[9] Knox D.L., "Inflammatory bowel disease," in THE EYE IN SYSTEMIC DISEASE, D.H. Gold and T.A. Weingeist, editors, J.B. Lippincott, Philadelphia, 1990, pp. 103.

[10] Sommer A., NUTRITIONAL BLINDNESS, Oxford University Press, 1982.

[11] Main A.N.H., et al, "Vitamin A deficiency in Crohn's disease," Gut 24: 1169-75, 1983.

[12] McClain C.J., Stuart M.A., "Zinc metabolism in the elderly," in GERIATRIC NUTRITION, John E. Morley, editor, Raven Press, New York, 1990.

[13] Werbach M.R., "Crohn's Disease," NUTRITIONAL INFLUENCES ON ILLNESS, Keats Publishing, New Canaan, CT., 1987, pp. 142-48.

[14] J. Pizzorno, M. Murray, "Crohn's Disease and Ulcerative Colitis," ENCYCLOPEDIA OF NATURAL MEDICINE, Prima Publishing, Rocklin, Ca., 1990, pp. 237-54.

[15] Williams J.M., O'Grady G.E., "Pancreatitis," in THE EYE IN SYSTEMIC DISEASE, D.H. Gold, T.A. Weingeist, editors, J.B. Lippincott, Philadelphia, 1990, pp. 106-08.

[16] Callaway W., Whitney C., SURVIVING WITH AIDS, Little Brown and Co., Boston, 1991.

[17] Russell R.M., "Gastrointestinal function and aging," in GERIATRIC NUTRITION, John E. Morley, editor, Raven Press, New York, 1990, pp. 232.

[18] Steinkuller P.G., "Hypovitaminoses and hypervitaminoses," in THE EYE IN SYSTEMIC DISEASE, J.B. Lippincott, Philadelphia, 1990, pp. 675-80.

[19] Schachat A.P., "Toxic and nutritional retionpathies," in RETINAL DYSTROPHIES AND DEGENERATIONS, D.A., Newsome, editor, Raven Press, New York, 1988, p. 351.

[20] Kellen R.I., Burde R.M., "Pernicious anemia," in THE EYE IN SYSTEMIC DISEASE, D.H. Gold, T.A. Weingeist, editors, J.B. Lippincott, Philadelphia, 1990, pp. 143.

[21] Mansfield J., ARTHRITIS THE ALLERGY CONNECTION, Thorsons, Britain, 1990.

[22] Murray M.T., THE HEALING POWER OF HERBS, Prima Publishing, Rocklin, CA., 1992.

[23] Bidlack W.R., "Nutritional requirements of the elderly," GERIATRIC NUTRITION, John E. Morley, editor, Raven Press, New York, 1990, pp. 41-72.

[24] Mitsuoka T., "Intentinal flora and aging," Nutrition Reviews, 50: 438-46, 1992.

[25] Whitney E.N., Hamilton E.M.N., Rolfes S.R., UNDERSTANDING NUTRITION, 5th edition, West Publishing Co., St. Paul, 1990, p. 482.

[26] Castleman M., THE HEALING HERBS, Rodale Press, Emmaus, PA, 1991.

INDEX

Note to Readers

If you have altered your diet or nutritional supplements, and you have experienced positive results, we would like to hear from you.

1. What type of eye problem do you have? (circle)

      CATARACTS   GLAUCOMA   MACULAR DEGENERATION
      DRY EYES   DIABETIC EYE PROBLEMS
      OTHER _____

2. Who diagnosed your eye condition?

      Optometrist? _____   Ophthalmologist? _____   Other _____

3. How long have you had this problem? _____

4. How long did it take before you experienced improvement? ___

5. If your vision improved, how would you explain it?

      Doctor said vision improved _____   Brighter vision__
      Better night vision _____   Better color vision _____
      Other _____

6. Are there activities you have been able to resume because of your improved sight? YES NO   Please list: _____

5. Had you tried nutritional or dietary programs previously?
      YES NO   Were they helpful? YES NO

6. What did you begin doing differently?

      Changed to low-fat diet _____   Began exercising _____
      Stopped smoking _____
      Began wearing UV-protective sunglasses _____
      Started taking nutritional supplements _____
      Which ones? (Please circle)
      OCUGUARD MAXILIFE   OCUDYNE OCUVITE
      OCUCARE OCUCAPS   VITAL EYEZ   SEE
      I-CAPS PLUS   NUTRIVISION   VIZION   CATA Rx
      OTHER _____

NAME _____

ADDRESS _____

CITY, STATE, ZIP _____

SEND TO HEALTH SPECTRUM PUBLISHERS
8851 Central Avenue, G-620, Montclair, CA. 91763

GIFT COPIES

Sent to your friends and loved ones,
So they can learn the secrets of good health and maintenance of sight.

HEALTH SPECTRUM PUBLISHERS

8851 Central Avenue, #G-620
Montclair, CA. 91763

Please send the following volumes of **NUTRITION AND THE EYES** to the address listed below, or a gift copy to the address in the adjacent box.

GIFT SHIPMENT TO:

_____
NAME
_____
STREET
_____
CITY
_____
STATE
_____
ZIP

A GIFT GREETING WILL BE ENCLOSED WITH YOUR ORDER IN THE NAME OF:
_____

☐ **Check box to order   VOLUME I**

Chapters cover the following topics: CATARACTS, PRESBYOPIA, MYOPIA, COMPUTER EYE STRAIN, BLEPHARITIS, EYELID SKIN CANCER, DROOPY EYELIDS, TRICHIASIS, OCULAR ROSACEA, BLEPHAROSPASM, DRY EYES, SJOGRENS' SYNDROME, KERATOCONUS, PTERYGIUM, CORNEA TRANSPLANT, EYE ALLERGY.

ISBN 1-885919-46-8   160 pages   **$24.50**

☐ **Check box to order   VOLUME II**

Chapters cover the following topics: MACULAR DEGENERATION, RETINITIS PIGMENTOSA, FLOATERS, RETINAL DETACHMENT, CIRCULATORY EYE DISORDERS, ARTIFICIAL SWEETENERS AND YOUR EYES, SMOKERS, SUNLIGHT-SUNGLASSES AND EYE HEALTH, DRUG SIDE EFFECTS, EYE PROBLEMS AND DIGESTIVE DISORDERS.

ISBN 1-885919-47-6   135 pages   **$24.50**

☐ **Check box to order   VOLUME III**

Chapters cover the following topics: GLAUCOMA, DIABETIC EYE DISEASE, MIGRAINE, UVEITIS, NIGHT VISION, HERPES EYE INFECTIONS, AIDS AND THE EYES, FOLK REMEDIES, DRIVING AND VISION

ISBN 1-885919-48-4   138 pages   **$24.50**

☐ **Check box to order   SUPPLEMENT**

Chapters cover the following topics: VITAMINS AND THE EYES, RESOURCES.

ISBN 1-885919-49-2 61 pages **$12.50**

☐ **Check box to order   ALL 3 VOLUMES**
Plus supplement
➡ Order as a set and save.
➡ ISBN 1-885919-45-X   **Total $59.50**

I am enclosing $_____ (plus $3.00 shipping & handling) per order. Send check or money order to HEALTH SPECTRUM PUBLISHERS. Add sales tax in Calif.

ORDERED BY:
NAME_____
STREET _____
CITY _____
STATE_____
ZIP _____
PHONE _____

Credit card orders

_____
CARD NUMBER
_____
SIGNATURE
_____
EXPIRATION DATE

Allow 4 weeks for delivery.   Add sales tax in California.
Add $3.00 shipping & handling per order (up to 4 books)

Receive the latest information about health, medicine, wellness and nutrition by subscribing to *"Here's To Your Health!"*

The monthly newsletter from the nationwide radio show with *Dr. Donald Carrow and Deborah Ray.*

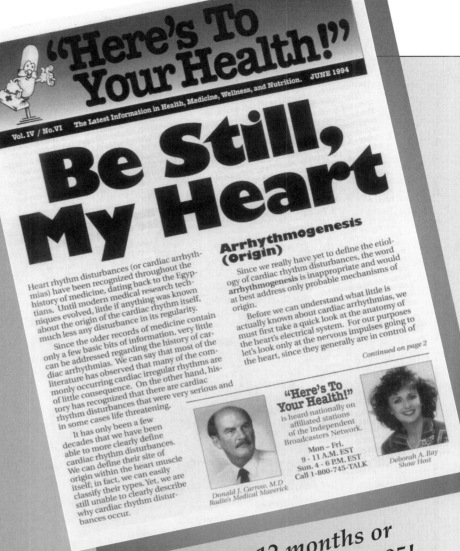

Just $37.95 for 12 months or two easy payments of $19.95!

SEND TO:

Here's To Your Health
PO BOX 130133
Tampa, Florida 33681

Or Call 1-800-283-1522 to order by telephone have your Mastercard and Visa ready.